THE ENERGIES
OF CROP CIRCLE

"To fly with Lucy Pringle over a crop circle formation, or walk carefully among the miraculously woven wheat, is up there with standing next to Spielberg during filming; she is an expert. These formations in our fields are the most enigmatic mystery of our day, and yet millions, who have never visited one, write them off with spoon-fed explanations. I have followed the phenomenon since the late eighties, visiting well over a dozen firsthand, once as the first visitor. No one has ever convinced me they were all created by the human hand. Lucy's exploration of the energy within the formations and its effect on our bodies is a particularly fascinating aspect of these beautiful messages in our fields. This is a book that will take you down many new and unexpected paths. A combination of compelling science and stories of extraordinary events recorded over a period of thirty years, this book lifts the crop circle phenomenon to previously unexplored levels of investigation, enhanced by Lucy's wonderful photography. A must-read for all travelers of the known and unknown."

SIR MARK RYLANCE, ACTOR, THEATER DIRECTOR, AND PLAYWRIGHT

"This book is a must for everyone interested in crop circles. It is well researched and proposes some fascinating new ideas that are sure to grab the attention of both the scientific and paranormal research communities. Crammed with captivating information, it makes compulsive reading."

GRAHAM PHILLIPS, AUTHOR OF *WISDOMKEEPERS OF STONEHENGE*

"For decades, crop circles have attracted the attention of scholars, photographers, hoaxers, and pranksters, making it difficult to understand the subject. Separating the wheat from the chaff can be difficult in such a mixed climate! Lucy Pringle and James Lyons separate fact from fiction, bringing a refreshing scientific approach to the hidden energies and dynamics of crop circles. The nature of consciousness, the ancient art of dowsing, and Earth Energies are explored in detail. The authors' research offers fascinating insights into the mesmerizing annual appearance of crop circles. The stunning photography drew me ever closer to the circles, and it felt like I was there. Enjoy this book, as it is a beacon of light that will illuminate your understanding of crop circles."

MARIA WHEATLEY, AUTHOR OF *DIVINING ANCIENT SITES*
AND PROFESSIONAL DOWSER

"For three decades, Lucy Pringle has been one of the most intrepid and persistent researchers of the mysterious crop circle phenomenon. In the face of often relentless skepticism or indifference from the mainstream, Lucy's passionate determination to focus on actual data, meticulously gathered from personal studies and the crucial testimony of many people, has enabled her to compile this very valuable book. Whatever anyone's opinions of where crop circles come from, the reality is that they have had a profound effect, both mentally and physically, on those who have visited them. *The Energies of Crop Circles* brilliantly records many of these experiences for future generations, who may one day, with advancing scientific discoveries, find a new context in which to place this intriguing evidence, which we dismiss at our peril."

ANDY THOMAS, MYSTERIES RESEARCHER
AND AUTHOR OF THE TRUTH AGENDA WEBSITE

"The combination of Lucy Pringle's elegant photographs and James Lyons's lucid explanations elevates *The Energies of Crop Circles* to a new understanding since the modern appearance of this ongoing fascinating and mysterious phenomenon. This is a book of value for everyone who seeks knowledge of our world."

MARCUS ALLEN, UK PUBLISHER OF *NEXUS MAGAZINE*

"Crop circles are fascinating, and this book allows us to explore the depth of our Universe and to receive new perceptions and knowledge, which is useful in this era of big changes."

LILOU MACÉ, AUTHOR OF *THE YONI EGG* AND HOST OF *LILOU MACÉ TV*

"The mysterious and often elaborate crop circles that have adorned the fields in southern England over the past 30 years have inspired the authors to make an in-depth study of people's experiences when visiting them. Lucy documents these fascinating accounts and, with the aid of scientist and dowser James Lyons, shows that the underlying science has a universal origin and intelligence. The selected circles are illustrated by Lucy's superb aerial photographs; relevant aspects of the science are detailed in the appendices."

ANDREW KING, PH.D., BIOLOGIST

"Not only is this a fascinating and entertaining book, but it is truly mind-expanding. The materialist paradigm, which permeates the science of today, finds us lacking in the conceptual equipment required to cope with the crop circle phenomenon. The accounts of people's experiences, reactions by animals, strange and meaningful synchronicities, and not least so many inexplicable facts on the ground, baffle the way of thinking that most of us have grown up with. It's no wonder why crop circles aren't featured in the mainstream media much—those writing about them don't know what to say!

James Lyons's comments are of great value. As he points out, earlier civilizations, and even tribal people today, have a conceptual map which can include such phenomena. His interpretation of crop circle geometry in relation to music is of special value.

This book should be widely read, especially by scientists."

ROGER TAYLOR, PH.D., B.V.SC., IMMUNOLOGIST

THE
ENERGIES
OF
CROP
CIRCLES

THE SCIENCE AND POWER OF A
MYSTERIOUS INTELLIGENCE

....

LUCY PRINGLE with JAMES LYONS

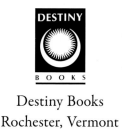

Destiny Books
Rochester, Vermont

Destiny Books
One Park Street
Rochester, Vermont 05767
www.DestinyBooks.com

Destiny Books is a division of Inner Traditions International

Library of Congress Cataloging-in-Publication Data
Names: Pringle, Lucy, author. | Lyons, James, (writer on dowsing), author.
Title: The energies of crop circles : the science and power of a mysterious
    intelligence / Lucy Pringle and James Lyons.
Description: Rochester, Vermont : Destiny Books, 2019. | Includes
    bibliographical references and index.
Identifiers: LCCN 2018038609 (print) | LCCN 2018056551 (ebook) |
    ISBN 9781620558676 (pbk.) | ISBN 9781620558683 (ebook)
Subjects: LCSH: Crop circles. | Healing. | Electromagnetic Fields—
    Physiological effect—Popular works.
Classification: LCC BL604.C5 P75 2019 (print) | LCC BL604.C5 (ebook) |
    DDC 001.94—dc23
LC record available at https://lccn.loc.gov/2018038609

Printed and bound in China by Reliance Printing Co., Ltd.

10   9   8   7   6   5   4   3   2

Text design and layout by Virginia Scott Bowman
This book was typeset in Garamond Premier Pro and Frutiger with Arquitecta used as the display typeface

To send correspondence to the author of this book, mail a first-class letter to the author c/o Inner Traditions • Bear & Company, One Park Street, Rochester, VT 05767, and we will forward the communication, or contact the author directly at **https://cropcircles.lucypringle.co.uk**.

CONTENTS

FOREWORD

by John Martineau

CROP CIRCLES ARE SOME of the most remarkable phenomena of our times. If they are paranormal then they are surely the most significant psychic events occurring today. If they are of alien origin then only fools would not pay them serious attention. If they are man-made, then they are probably the best-known modern art in the world, as people recognize them from Moscow to Tokyo—beat that, Damien Hirst!

I spent four or five very happy summers crop circling (yes it's a verb) in the early 1990s. As database manager for the Centre for Crop Circle Studies I had a mobile phone the size of a large brick and drove around visiting crop formations collecting information, making surveys, and meeting people. And what wonderful people I met. In the middle of the night in one formation I met an Alaskan scientist who was convinced that crop circles were the past imprints of future power stations. In another I met a writer who was sure that they were messages from the collective subconscious executed by fairies. In another I met a psychic who regularly communicated with alien spacecraft, and who could summon balls of light. I spent nights manning infra-red microwave plasma scanning equipment for a team from the University of Tokyo. One fine morning I met a couple who had just seen an enormous flying saucer covered with lights, which had created a crop circle, before flying off. I spoke to five other people who had seen it before a man from the Ministry of Defense confiscated my report. It was like being in the middle of the X-files. And, right in the middle of all the intrigue, I met Lucy Pringle, and later, Jim Lyons.

I was immediately fascinated by what Lucy was doing. Like her and Jim, I was talking to a lot of people, and kept hearing the same stories. By far the most common subject of conversation, aside from who or what was making crop circles, was the extraordinary effect they seemed to have on people visiting them. Cameras jammed. Batteries suddenly ran down. Strange buzzing noises were recorded. People returned to their cars and found they wouldn't start. Or they bumped into close friends they hadn't seen for years or just random people from the same distant village or with the same professions or names. Crop circles seemed connected to some higher reality. Some people started having visions, seeing auras, or experienced extraordinary healing. People felt elated. People felt puzzled. People felt peculiar.

Some people felt happy-peculiar, I certainly did. Going into a fresh crop circle at dawn made my fingers tingle and the hair on the back of my neck stand up. With a group of friends we would slowly crawl inch by inch over the dew-coated swirled wheat, lifting it up and looking for footprints, crushed clods of earth beneath, or any other evidence of humans in there before us, and find none. Other people, however, would visit a crop formation and immediately feel uncomfortable, discombobulated, and then develop a headache, either immediately or half an hour after leaving. Many people felt intensely sleepy soon after visits to crop circles. They would have to pull over and snooze and often reported life-changing dreams.

Lucy's work, collected in this excellent book and illustrated with her masterful photographs, demonstrates the extraordinary range of psychological and physiological responses people have had to crop circles. Running alongside this exposition, Jim Lyons's meticulous scientific research provides some fascinating and thought-provoking explanations of what really might be going on.

Crop circles are ephemeral—here today, gone tomorrow. All that remains of them after they are harvested each year are the photographs and stories told by people who visited them. This book is the first detailed collection of such stories, and it represents an important milestone in crop circle research. The photographic record may tell us a certain amount about this extraordinary phenomenon, but these stories, carefully collected over the past thirty years, and many reproduced here for the first time, tell us much more. I can't personally vouch for every story in this book, but I can vouch for hundreds of other similar ones I heard myself from complete strangers. What this book reveals is a far more nuanced, complex, and intelligent phenomenon than many will have suspected.

An old Chinese proverb says: Mind, like parachute, works best when open. Holding that in mind, please read on . . .

JOHN MARTINEAU is publisher and editor of the international award-winning Wooden Books pocket liberal arts series, which has been translated into 20 languages worldwide. He is the author of *A Little Book of Coincidence in the Solar System* and *Mazes and Labyrinths in Great Britain* and the editor of *Megalith: Studies in Stone.*

ACKNOWLEDGMENTS

OVER THE PAST ALMOST THIRTY YEARS I have had the pleasure and privilege of meeting and chatting with hundreds of people both inside and outside the crop circles, in person, or by email and letter. I have been inspired by their stories and sometimes even moved to tears by their experiences and how the crop circles have impacted and changed their lives in often unexpected and wonderful ways. There can be no doubting the veracity of their experiences as they have frequently happened so unexpectedly that people have been totally taken aback by what has taken place and still can hardly believe how their thinking and being have been changed completely and opened up as a result. New realms of understanding have entered their lives, giving them changed and broadened perspectives. Some of the reports I have received are confidential and will always remain so, but others have gladly shared their stories, and I would like to thank all those who have played an essential part in this book—each one imparting his or her own precious pearl of wisdom.

Writing this book has reminded me of many of my own experiences, which, like others, have happened literally out of the blue, some good, some bad. These have given me insights into previously unexplored regions of my being and my understanding of our world, my fellow beings, and our planet and often other unseen worlds. They have all been part of my journey, a journey of exploration and further learning.

Even though writing has always been an essential part of my being ever since I can first remember, it essentially is a lonely yet fascinating experience requiring much exhilarating research but also strict discipline. As a result it may seem to be a selfish occupation, and so I would like to thank my many friends and family, whom I may have neglected, for their patience and understanding.

However, my most grateful and enormous thanks and gratitude must be reserved for Patricia Daubncy, without whose encouragement this book would never have happened. I had started writing it and it was largely finished—at which point the wastepaper basket seemed the most fitting place for it. Patricia thought otherwise and persuaded me to continue. Reluctantly I consented and asked James Lyons, my longtime friend and colleague, if he would contribute his wisdom. He gladly agreed and so the fate of the book was sealed. Patricia has never failed to give unstintingly of her time and encouragement throughout, with endless patience and wonderful good humor in helping pull the book into shape. She has played a major role. James Lyons is in full agreement with this and adds his most grateful thanks to Patricia for all her invaluable help.

LUCY PRINGLE

AN EXCITING AND CHALLENGING JOURNEY

by Lucy Pringle

True wisdom comes to each of us when we realize how little we understand about life, ourselves, and the world around us.

SOCRATES (CA. 469–399 BCE)

THE TITLE OF THIS BOOK IS *The Energies of Crop Circles,* so we must ask the question, "Is this really so?" "Do crop circles actually have mysterious energies?" And further, "Can these energies heal us?" The answer to these questions is "Yes." Having had an unexpected personal healing experience in 1990, and having had many others reported to me, I am left with no other option than to say, "Yes, it does happen."

How did I first get interested in the subject of crop circles? It all happened when my two children left the nest and suddenly there was a terrible bottomless void in my life, known as the empty nest syndrome. After years of bringing up the boys I found I had time for myself, and I could either sink or swim. What was I going to do with this new syndrome of wondering how was I going to fill my days, and what was I going to do with my time?

At that time I had just recently moved to Hampshire, and I suddenly found myself in the place where the early crop circles first appeared right on my very doorstep. This started a new and unexpected chapter in my life, one in which I have been increasingly involved for over a quarter of a century.

When I was asked to write a book about healing in crop circles, I never realized what an exciting and challenging journey I was about to take. I was a founding member of the first academic society to study the circles, the Centre for Crop Circle Studies, set up at Easter 1990, so I have been there from the beginning. I have seen our understanding of the circles progress beyond all recognition as the technology and methodology for studying them have improved and evolved.

As so often happens, despite remaining a group for many years, we all individually seemed to find our own particular lines of research. I fell into mine purely by chance one gloriously sunny day in July 1990, three months after the society was set up.

A GOOD PLACE

I would like to tell you about what happened in a crop circle in the Winchester area on that day in July 1990. I had my sister, Amanda Spence, and a close mutual friend, Maggie Randall, with me. The latter had the great misfortune to suffer from Raynaud's phenomenon, a condition affecting blood circulation. We went into the crop circle, and I proceeded in my usual way recording the YIN and YANG energies (YIN and YANG represent the Female and Male energies, respectively, and can be detected by dowsing) and noting the strength of the different energy forces, as well as the manner and direction in which the crop lay. Having almost completed this, I sat down on a strong energy point on the perimeter of the YANG circle with great relief as I had hurt my right shoulder playing a ferocious set of mixed tennis doubles the previous evening. I had been unable to use my right hand to brush my teeth that evening, as the pain in raising my arm was considerable.

As I was sitting, relaxing in the circle, I became aware of energy rippling through my shoulders. I gently moved my right shoulder and found to my amazement that I could move it without pain. I stayed where I was and let the energy continue to flow until my shoulder was completely mobile and free of pain. Having been full of doom and gloom at the prospect of being out of tennis for the rest of the season, I was joyful at my recovery.

What happened to my friend was no less dramatic; on becoming aware of what was happening to me, I called to her and suggested she should come and sit close by me. I did not tell her what had happened to me; I simply suggested she might find it a "good place" to sit. She immediately expressed a feeling of tremendous well-being and said her fingers were tingling. She later described it this way: "I can't explain the tingling I experienced in my fingertips except to say it was as if my fingers had been cold, as in a Raynaud's spasm, and that they were warming up, that is, the blood was beginning to flow properly again. But my fingers had not been cold—quite the opposite when one remembers that that Sunday was probably one of the hottest days of the summer!" I still had a few things I wanted to check in the configuration so I left her there, and when I returned found her lying happily on her side with a blissful smile on her face. This she cannot normally do, for as she says,

It is rare that Raynaud's phenomenon (or syndrome) is an "illness" by itself. Usually there is an underlying cause, and in my case it is scleroderma. Scleroderma, in turn, can be of two types—either morphea, which is localized, or systemic sclerosis (which is what I have)—and can affect different organs. One of the commonest organs to be affected is the esophagus; the sphincter muscle to the stomach becomes slack and consequently allows the stomach acids to flow up, thus causing ulcers which, when healed, form strictures and thereby narrow the pipe. This is why I have trained myself to lie propped up; otherwise it is like having perpetual heartburn! And I didn't get "heartburn" when lying flat in the crop circle!

She was most reluctant to leave the circle after lying on her side for at least twenty minutes. Sadly she is now deceased as a result of a different condition, but I remained in touch with her regularly after that day, and she became accustomed to her newfound sense of well-being. She was sleeping extremely well and her energy increased noticeably, and, in general, there was a continued marked improvement in her condition.

After my own personal healing experience in 1990, I realized that there must be many other people experiencing similar effects, and, in order to try and explore what was happening, I drew up a rudimentary questionnaire to find out more. I was amazed by the huge response.

This extraordinary event was the trigger point and catalyst for my years of research into what has now become increasingly sophisticated and scientific work. This work has involved many wonderful people who have contributed unstintingly to my somewhat seemingly "way out" ideas that have, nevertheless, produced significant results and taken me further down the path of investigation. To my amazement I was once told that, as I was describing an idea, I had in fact unwittingly described a certain complex theorem. I have to thank the genes from my father's side, as members of his family were all brilliant scientists, whereas I had no scientific training and have now come in at post-grad level without any training but with strong gut feelings!

James Lyons, my coauthor and a polymath in his own right, has been one of those leading lights who unreservedly have given me their time and encouragement, as he too came to understand the results we were finding in the crop circles were all part of a far greater compass of learning and discovery. Lyons is a chartered engineer specializing in aeronautical and electrical engineering. He had a long and successful career in the aerospace industry and academia. His enthusiasm is catching, and to work with him is a delight.

This book will lead you along our paths of adventure as we seek to shed more light on this brain-rattling and wonderful subject. When approaching this subject, it may be best to fasten your seat belts!

THE CREATION
OF CROP CIRCLES

by James Lyons

WHEN WE LOOK AT the formation of crop circles we need to start with our Solar System. The Sun is the key energy source, which is electrically charged like the positive terminal of a battery. It emits particles incessantly, and this emission is called the "solar wind."

At the moment the Sun has on its surface black-looking features from which spiraling tubes of energy are emitted. These are so-called torsion waves because of their essentially twisting nature. These waves strike the magnetosphere, which surrounds the Earth and is a layer of charged particles supported there by the Earth's magnetic field. This layer occasionally breaks down and lets through these Sun waves.

The waves mainly enter the Earth via the poles, which give rise to the aurora borealis at the North Pole and the aurora australis at the South Pole. When the waves break through at other points around the Earth they give rise to very high-altitude plasma effects known as "sprites." All of this is the source of the electric charge we find around the Earth. The Earth is negatively charged and acts like the other terminal of a battery.

The charge within the Earth is arranged into patterns like cymatic patterns of sand on a vibrating drum surface. The key structures are north-south, east-west grid patterns, which we detect as ley lines, to use the older terminology.

These are the "graph paper" on which crop circles are created. The formations consist of mostly six rings and eight radial patterns. The geometry is governed by the diatonic scale, but we need not go further at this juncture on this very important topic. These nodal points of the rings and the radial lines are found in all ancient sites around the world and in churches built before the Reformation. These web patterns are the result of combinations of the telluric currents and the water streams beneath the ground. The water is, of course, electrically charged.

We need now to consider cloud formations, which are also made of water droplets, all charged, that cluster together. If the weather pressure pattern is of a certain kind, then the clouds' electric positive charge engages with the negative charge of the Earth below. This forms an enormously strong electric field, which, not surprisingly, creates a discharge to ground.

It strikes at the point of lowest resistance, which is the center of the Earth's "acupuncture point," or, more precisely, the water-stream crossover point. The water breaks down into gaseous form, hydrogen and oxygen. Like a smoker blowing a smoke ring or a dolphin blowing a ring, the toroidal ring formed, being now less dense than its surroundings, rises like a bubble in a bottle. It breaks through the ground into the crop from below and, because it is at a lower pressure than the ambient air pressure, there is an enormous sucking down process, which is responsible for flattening the crop.

The wave-type nature of the toroidal ring possesses spirals on its surface, which are responsible for flattening the crop in very characteristic ways. The initial lightning strike has already broken down the local air into nitrogen and oxygen, which interpenetrates with the crop and recombines to enhance the nitrate level.

This is a simple description for the creation of crop circles.

However the dramatic changes in mainstream science are again revealing the concept of Cosmic Consciousness. Crop circle investigators are confirming that the human mind operates synonymously with the Crop Circle Consciousness. This is our link to the crop circle phenomenon.

1

SANCTITY
WITHIN THE CIRCLES

If the doors of perception were cleansed everything would appear to man as it is, infinite.

WILLIAM BLAKE (1757–1827)

OCCASIONALLY, PERMANENT HEALING can occur as a result of visiting crop circles, but the majority of reports fall into the negative list of effects: visitors to crop circles automatically expect to feel well and therefore are surprised and dismayed when the opposite occurs (and as a result will submit a negative report, whereas a beneficial experience unless strikingly unusual will be accepted as being normal).

However, while the greater number of healing events are unfortunately only temporary in nature, they are still worth discussing in order to illustrate the effects of the inherent residual "energies" and their subsequent impact on living systems, even from a distance.

Arthritis and rheumatism sufferers seem to gain noticeable but temporary relief. Longtime sufferer Leslie Clementson is one of my most generous reporters:

After doing a night watch on Knapp Hill, near Alton Barnes, we drove as far as we could and then walked the rest of the way, and as before I was in a lot of pain when we reached it. We were meeting friends who had walked up; we wandered around it for a while then stopped in the center for about

1

fifteen minutes. Unlike the Lockeridge, near Marlborough, formation (1992) when the swelling in my feet was so drastically reduced that my shoes kept falling off, I was unaware of anything happening until we started to walk back to the car only to discover that I could almost keep up with Steve. I haven't been able to do that since Lockeridge. It's a shame it did not help Steve, who has a broken toe!

I received a further report from Leslie dated September 7, 2001, saying,

I thought I would let you know that the healing I received in the Milk Hill formation, near Devizes, is just starting to subside. It lasted longer than the Lockeridge one. I now look forward to the next.

And she sent a further report from a different visit to the same formation some years later:

I had been having problems with very painful and swollen feet for about ten days and had difficulty getting to the formation, even though it was a relatively short distance from my car. When I was inside the formation, I felt no pain at all and could walk without difficulty. Once I was a few yards down the tramline again the discomfort returned.

Was this due to the uneven ground? But when she visited the East Field formation on July 12, 2007,

with some difficulty walking and with additional pain in one shoulder, once inside the formation, both feet and shoulder became pain free, and discomfort then returned soon after leaving the formation. Obviously the shoulder pain was not related to the soft surface, so it seems that it was being in the formation that gave relief. I have visited other formations this year, but no others have affected pain levels.

Diana Cussons, a dear friend of over eighty years old, suffering from severe osteoporosis, had long beseeched me to take her into a formation to experience the "energies." Her stipulations were it had to be one that was new, one that was close to where she lived, and one that was fairly near to the road so that she would not have too far to walk. It just happened that one appeared nearby

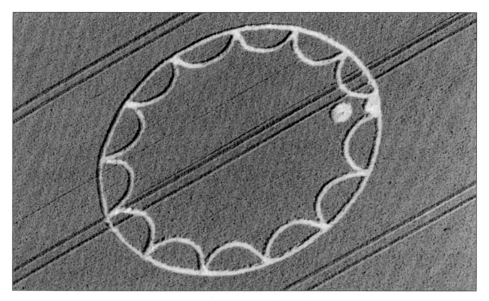

Fig. 1.1. Pastry Cutter, Teglease Down, East Meon, Hampshire, June 30, 1997.

at Teglease Down, East Meon, Hampshire, on June 30, 1997, a circle within easy reach of the car, which meant she would not have too far to walk before reaching the circle.

I had found a formation that seemed to fit the bill. "Was 6:00 a.m. too early?" "Not a bit, how about 5:00 a.m.?" she replied. We settled on 6:00 a.m. It was an overcast, heavily clouded but sultry morning as we made our way into the field and walked toward the formation following the tramline, the lines used by farmers in order to facilitate crop sowing and spraying, Diana coming at her own pace using her walking stick. What was a short walk for me was quite another thing for her. At this time of day there is a certain indescribable magic about. The birds and animals treat you as one of them, there is no fear, for we are all part of the same ecological system, all interdependent and interactive.

The ground was wet, covered in heavy overnight dew, so sitting down in the circle was out of the question. Time speeds up in genuine formations, and one hour can seem like thirty minutes. We didn't talk a lot, there seemed to be an overwhelming sense of awe as though in a cathedral, and silence was appropriate.

The quietness of mind and spirit one experiences is memorable; there is a sense of total security, and in that silence and safety one allows oneself to transcend to higher levels of consciousness.

I dropped Diana home by 8:00 a.m. Two hours later she telephoned in great excitement: she was totally free of pain. Normally after such strenuous exercise she would have been flat on her back in bed, suffering immense pain. Over a month later she was still free of pain.

WONDERFUL BUT TEMPORARY

Another old friend, Christina Thistlethwayte, reluctantly came with me to a crop circle at King's Somborne, Hampshire, in 2011. Her reluctance was due to the fact that she had an agonizingly painful back and polymyalgia rheumatica (a muscular condition of unknown cause that can be so painful that people sometimes find themselves unable to get out of bed in the morning). However, she managed to hobble into the formation.

There were several others in the circle and we chatted, and I walked around examining the lay of the crop. (It had formed on a rainy night but photographs taken early the following morning showed no trace of mud on the fallen crop, which would have been present if people walking round with boards had flattened the crop.)

Suddenly the sky appeared threatening, and we walked back to the car. As we were getting in, Christina announced, "All the pain in my back has

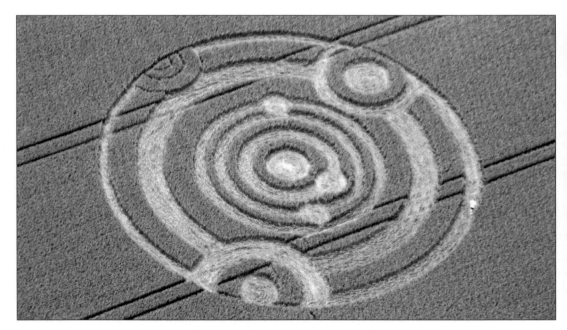

Fig. 1.2. King's Somborne, Hampshire, June 18, 2011.

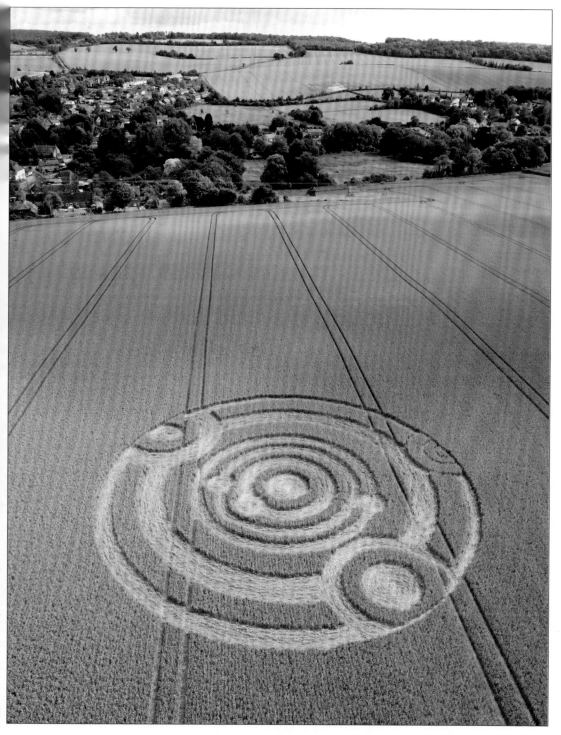

Fig. 1.3. King's Somborne, Hampshire, within the larger landscape,
June 18, 2011.

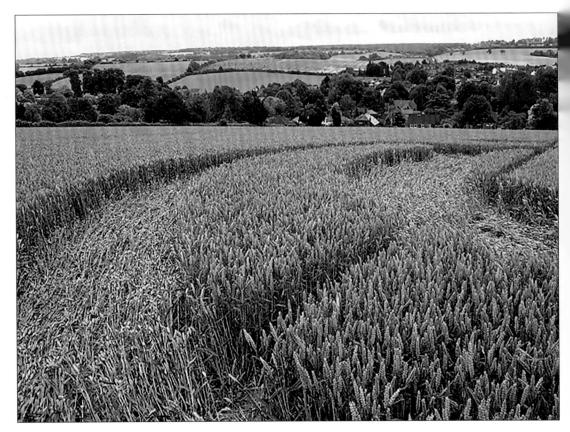

Fig. 1.4. A ground-level view at King's Somborne, Hampshire, June 18, 2011.

gone!" Wonderful, but so often it is only temporary, and I told her that it might not last.

As I dropped her home, to my astonishment she stood on one leg and brought her knee up to her chin and then repeated it with the other leg! Amazed, I tried it myself on returning home. Fine if you are fit, but not easy if you are in any pain. She had no pain for four days. What a blessed respite!

A BEDTIME BLESSING

Yet another report from a now-deceased elderly lady, Dorothy Colles, who suffered from both arthritis and macular degeneration (an eye condition whereby sight becomes increasingly limited). She was possessed of a penetratingly clear mind, and during the Second World War worked in photographic intelligence in the Middle East.

We entered the 1999 Warnford, Hampshire, formation on a sunny day in

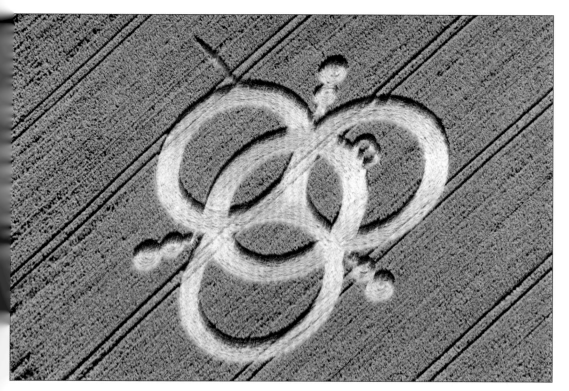

Fig. 1.5. Warnford Knot, Warnford, Hampshire, July 20, 1999.

July. Dorothy and I walked slowly round the formation, examining the general layout but, as so often happens, the desire to sit quietly and meditate was overwhelming.

Dorothy immediately knew exactly where she wanted to sit. "You will have to pull me up later," she announced.

I went to an area close by and sank into a deep meditation. After what seemed like a short time (but was in fact thirty minutes) Dorothy's head suddenly appeared over the top of the standing crop. No help had been needed—there she was, standing upright, having shot up like a cork out of a champagne bottle!

Dorothy recounts her visit thus:

This was the first formation I had ever been in . . . first impression was of an affectionate amused sense of "welcome" from the image to me. I was struck with wonder. There was a feeling of Presence—wholly benign. When I lay down on the laid corn there was an uprush of security and assurance that was amazing, and as I stroked the horizontal layering it felt as responsive as a family animal, a pony, a Labrador, or whatever—it was familiar not strange.

I got up without the usual arthritic creaks and effort without even noticing and left the beautiful quadruple rings with regret. I would have liked to stay all day there with them and that all-encompassing friendliness. There was no sense of time.

I am eighty-two and have collected several impediments along the way, but none of this seemed relevant while we were there. Afterward the energy bubbled up in everyday life. When I go to bed I deliberately relive the moment of walking in and lying down and that initial delight before I sleep—it's a bedtime blessing.

A FORM OF REJUVENATION?

Another delightful account came from an intrepid participant in one of my crop circle tours. Nearly eighty, Doreen Binks was originally concerned that she would not have the energy or stamina to last the day of vigorous walking, most demanding of which was the mile-plus trek in the afternoon (having already visited two formations in the morning) up to the 2009 Ogbourne St. Andrew "Trilobite," near Marlborough, Wiltshire, walking zigzag along the bottom of the field and then up a long uphill and twisty side tramline in order to reach the formation.

However, her glowing report tells me,

I felt tired as we reached the Ogbourne Maisie crop circle and sat down in the circle for about ten minutes—on leaving the site, I was surprised to find that my fatigue had gone. As we reached Stonehenge I was anticipating feeling tired, having been on the go all day. I leaned against the stones and felt only a small tingle in one hand, but on leaving the site, I found I was no longer tired on arriving home at 10:00 p.m.! I was feeling refreshed and not hungry. I had the best night's sleep in months, and the following day woke up feeling very calm and positive, which lasted all day. I was apprehensive about how I would cope with a fourteen-hour day; so the outcome was a big surprise—something happened—what? Can one tap into this form of rejuvenation?

One woman who had recently had a hip operation found that by simply looking at a formation from nearby, she was able to walk a distance that the previous day had been quite beyond her capability and was beyond the laws of probability. Many people have remarked on a new outer clarity of vision

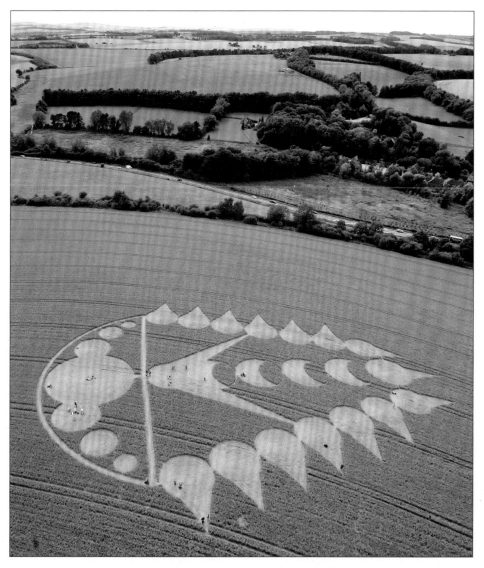

Fig. 1.6. Ogbourne St. Andrew,
within larger landscape, Wiltshire, July 29, 2009.

as though the scenery is made up of sharply defined "cutouts." A new inner clearness of vision is also often reported.

HOT FEET

Dan Voice, a landscape gardener, had been suffering from a groin strain for five to six days prior to our expedition and was in some pain. As we were walking

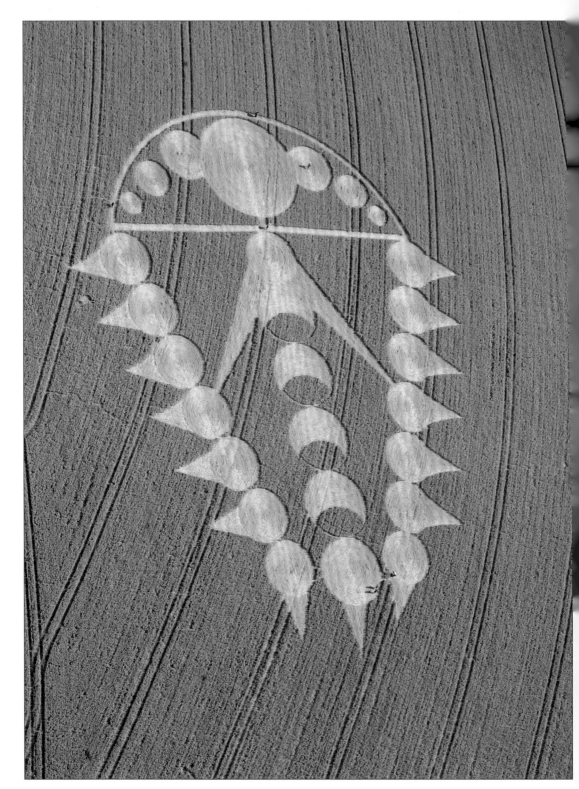

Fig. 1.7. Ogbourne St. Andrew, Wiltshire,
July 29, 2009.

in the tramline toward the formation, he suddenly stopped and called out to me. He looked ecstatic and said he had never ever experienced such a feeling of happiness and peace, almost beyond words. "At the same time the soles of my feet began to warm. The discomfort in my groin disappeared. The warming of my feet became intense but not painful."

Another report of "hot feet" was sent to me by someone visiting the Barbury Castle "Flower" in Wroughton. She experienced "warmth on the bottom of my feet, heaviness lying down, increased sense of smell and general awareness." On both occasions the weather was cool and cloudy.

What possible explanation could there be? We know that subtle energies and eddy currents in the brain kick-start the hypothalamus. Two of the effects are increased thirst and sense of smell. Also, in Dan's case, the nerves running down his leg were stimulated. This often occurs to people who have suffered some sort of spinal trauma, are diabetic, or have arthritis.

The hypothalamus is a very important part of the forebrain, which lies below the thalamus, and forms the lower part of the ventricle and its floor. Its integrity is essential to life, for it is concerned with the "vegetative" functions. It plays a major part in regulating the temperature of the body, body weight and appetite, sexual behavior and rhythms, blood pressure and fluid balance, and can even be said to be the physical basis of the emotions.

We need to examine the possible reason for these encouraging reactions. We do not know enough about the "cause" of rheumatism or arthritis, but we do know the effect is inflammation. Could the residual effects of the electro-magnetic fields present in some formations be acting as an anti-inflammatory? We are told that there are over a hundred types of arthritis, including osteoarthritis and gout. The word *arthritis* means "joint inflammation." Inflammation is one of the body's natural reactions to disease or injury and includes swelling, pain, and stiffness. Inflammation that lasts for a very long time or recurs, as in arthritis, can lead to tissue damage.

Rheumatoid arthritis is an autoimmune disease. With this condition, some-thing seems to trigger the immune system to attack the joints and sometimes other organs of the body. The exact cause of rheumatoid arthritis is unknown, but it is thought to be due to a combination of genetic, environmental, and hormonal factors. Other theories suggest that a virus or bacteria may alter the immune system, causing it to attack the joints.

NO BUMP!

Some reports, however, seem to go beyond medical and scientific explanation and take us into areas as yet little understood or explored.

There is a consciousness present in everything around us, the "Gaia" consciousness as described by James Lovelock, and in genuine crop circle formations, owing to their very size and complexity, there is evidence of an additional intelligence, intent, and focusing.

A now-deceased old friend, Colette Ardagh, after visiting the Corhampton circle in Hampshire in 2001, had an extraordinary cure. Shortly before our visit, Colette had broken her collarbone and was still receiving regular physical therapy.

While in the field I had asked everyone to collect a few stones as markers, for use in marking out certain areas for further research, without thinking that Colette might have a problem. To her amazement she was able to stretch out her damaged shoulder quite easily to pick up the stones.

A few days later she attended her physical therapy appointment. Her regular physiotherapist was on holiday, so she was seen by a replacement physiotherapist who, on examining her shoulder, looked puzzled and asked Colette if she had really broken her collarbone since the usual bump (there for life) marking where the bone mends was not present! The physiotherapist was astonished, as she had never seen this effect before.

In 2011 Jackie Faulkner, one of my volunteers for our scientific research day in July, had long suffered from a sore bunion and had difficulty walking any distance. Returning home after being inside the circle at Barbury Castle, Wiltshire, she found to her amazement that the bunion had diminished in size, and the skin was loose and flabby instead of tightly stretched. A bunion is painful: it is a bony deformity of the joint at the base of the big toe, known as the metatarsophalangeal joint. Sadly the reduction was only temporary, but one has to ask—how can a bony structure reduce in size even for a short period of time?

I COULDN'T SLEEP BECAUSE
OF THE PAIN IN MY NECK

Sadly, it is not possible to follow up on every case to establish if the cure has been permanent. However, I would like to present two cases of permanent healing to date.

Steve Meredith sent me a fascinating report, which needs further investigation.

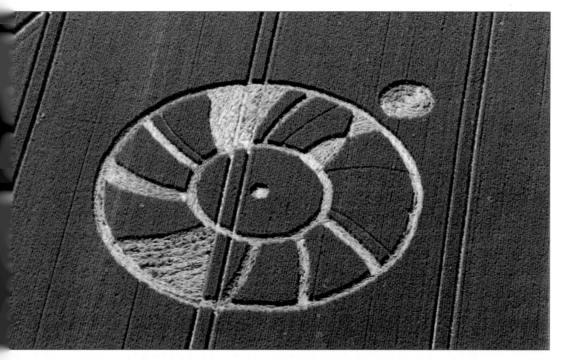

Fig. 1.8. Corhampton, Hampshire, June 18, 2001.

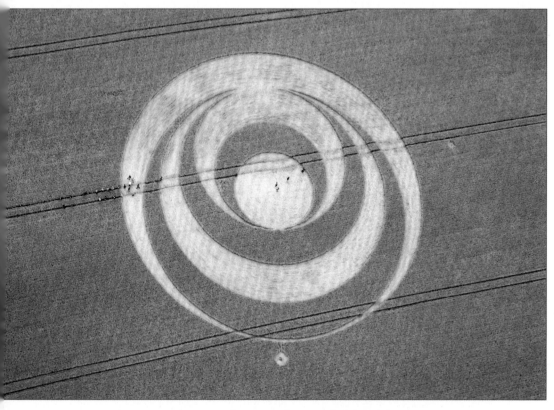

Fig. 1.9. Barbury Castle, Wroughton, Wiltshire, July 2, 2011.

He told me that he had had a bad waterskiing accident in his youth. He had pulled muscles badly in his neck but recovered well. About ten years later he started to suffer increasingly bad neck pains that were diagnosed as arthritis. By the summer of 2009, he was finding it hard to get any sleep at night.

In August 2009 he and his wife took their caravan to Wiltshire. Being in the caravan he found it even more difficult to get any sleep and could only do so by using a special pillow and lying on one side of his head.

While in Wiltshire they visited several crop circles in the Marlborough area, about twelve or thirteen in all, but it was during his visit to the "Hummingbird" formation at Stanton St. Bernard, Milk Hill, that he realized that the pains in his neck had completely disappeared.

> I am 99.5 percent free of pain. I get the odd tingle now and then. In the days leading up to that day I was in terrible pain and could hardly sleep at night, but the evening after we went in I was free of pain. The relief was tremendous and this continued for several months with only the occasional twinge until after a flight to Antigua and back, when they returned noticeably.

I have been in touch with him regularly since then, and he tells me that his neck is still 70 percent better than it had been prior to his visit to the "Hummingbird."

Many people are researching the damaging effects of radio masts; also there is a growing amount of literature and research into the beneficial properties of pulsed electromagnetic fields (EMFs).

Milk Hill, at 295 meters (968 feet), is one of the highest points for some miles. This is relevant as Steve Meredith and his wife were staying in an aluminum-walled caravan, which would concentrate the signals. Possibly a standing wave developed in which he slept. Could it be that the combination of frequency, amplitude, and pulse rate with rise and fall time of the signals did the trick?

I WAS NO LONGER HOBBLING

The next report comes from Sue Bowness. In 2010 she went on the Glastonbury Symposium crop circle tour but with damaged hamstrings she was not hopeful of being able to walk any distance into a crop circle. The coach stopped at the Vernham Dean formation, Hampshire, and Sue hobbled up the field into the circle.

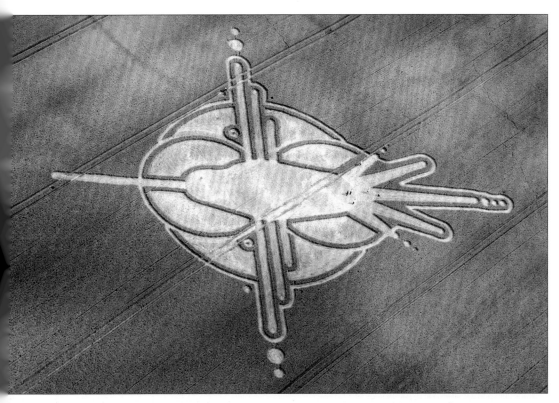

Fig. 1.10. The Hummingbird, Stanton St. Bernard, Milk Hill, Wiltshire, July 2, 2009.

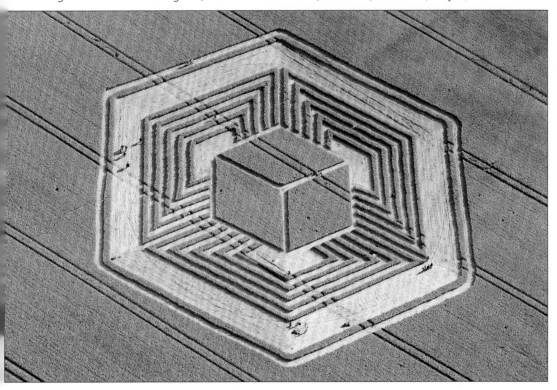

Fig. 1.11. Vernham Dean, Fosbury, Hampshire, July 17, 2010.

At the time of the tour I had damaged hamstrings in both legs stemming from December 2009 and was walking unevenly and had had an aching neck for two weeks.

As soon as I reached the road (after visiting the formation) and took a few strides, I realized I was no longer hobbling but walking evenly, with my stride lengthened to what it had been before the injuries. I felt rebalanced. The dizziness and aching neck persisted for another two weeks or so but are now gone.

I have been in regular touch with Sue, and she tells me the cure has indeed been maintained.

There is often an extraordinary feeling of sanctity within the circles; it reminds one of the wondrous cathedral at Chartres, and one feels overcome with awe and wonderment. I find this experience incredibly humbling, as though I have been touched by the Hand of God, and as is the case when treading on consecrated ground, one must behave accordingly, treating the moment with reverence. It is an experience one never forgets; it is as though for one brief period of time you are a flame within the Flame, having risen beyond the fetters of earthly constraints. I call it the "cathedral effect."

A wonderful sense of "Oneness" is often experienced. This can also be shown as a spike in the brain stem of between 18 and 18.5 Hz. This is the threshold of the three major sensory systems: sight, sound, and touch.

THE CATHEDRAL EFFECT

On entering the formation I felt a strong, warm inner glow, accompanied by high-frequency sounds around my head. I felt a little weakness in my legs, which has happened before in crop circles. I felt drawn to talk to people and found the unusually high level of openness that I have often experienced with people in crop circles in the past. To me, this is a real contrast to normal everyday life wherein people don't really communicate; they are so busy just living their roles day to day in a rather isolated existence. The crop formations seem to bring everything out of people that would not normally be discussed in everyday life. There was a remarkably joyous feeling of "Oneness" with the Universe.

Other reports tell us:

- "I felt peaceful, blissful and close to God, so I sat for a long time and meditated."
- "Experienced tingling sensations in my legs. I sat and meditated in the green center on the apex and felt a tremendous sense of well-being and an elongation of the spine. Breathing out, I descended down a pole toward the center of the Earth, inhaling as I went up the pole into an infinite Universe. Because I had tight muscles in my neck from the airplane flight, I lay down and positioned my neck right over the center apex, a fulcrum of energy, and relaxed and felt the muscle spasm melt into relaxation. It was just a wonderful experience."
- "Emotionally charged *and* felt an intense sense of love-impersonal which lasted about an hour."
- "I had an overwhelming feeling of vastness, wonder, and love—like things I had known deep within about other states of consciousness and dimensions were real."

I will close this chapter with a lovely story about my favorite 2014 circle, which appeared on July 8 at Tetbury Lane, near Charlton in Wiltshire. Despite the farmer refusing admission, it graced the landscape for several weeks.

It was a geometrically harmonious formation made up of a tripod of small triangles inside a broken triangle, which in turn was surrounded by a broken circle (see pages 18 and 19).

It seems that the young owner-farmer was not getting on all that well with his girlfriend at the time—that is until they visited the circle one glorious, warm, sunny evening, and all their differences were resolved.

Circles can unexpectedly work their magic.

COMMENTS BY JAMES LYONS

With this background we are now in a position to address the key issue of this book—how does all this energy result in healing?

The origins of the vibrational approach to healing have a long history, going back at least to the Yogic Period in India around 6000 BCE. It is well accepted in both esoteric scenarios and mainstream physics that the Cosmos is pervaded by a variety of cyclical processes. Everyone, even from a young

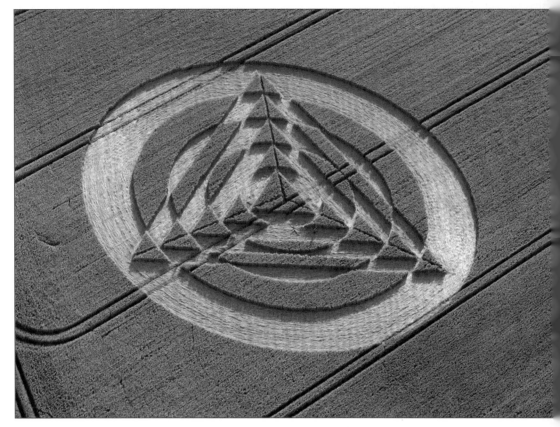

Fig. 1.12. Tetbury Lane, near Charlton, Wiltshire. Reported July 8, 2014.
A tripod of small triangles inside a broken triangle, which, in turn,
is surrounded by a broken circle. Barley, approx. 130-feet diameter.
(See fig. 1.13 for a view of the circle within the larger landscape.)

age, is aware of our day-night cycle. Such a process, due of course to Earth rotation, defines our clock cycle. Likewise, we have our annual cycle and, even more abstruse, there is the Mayan Galactic Cycle. In other words, the whole Cosmos is cyclical. We are just beginning to comprehend that frequencies of all kinds, having been the basis of cosmic structure, have in due course filtered down to living matter, which may not be unique in the Cosmos but, beyond Earth, appears to be rare.

Everyone soon comprehends that if something is vibrating strongly then nearby objects vibrate in harmony with this source. This is termed "forced or induced vibration." Although many people have encountered the phenomenon, the idea that living matter may also vibrate in sympathy with its

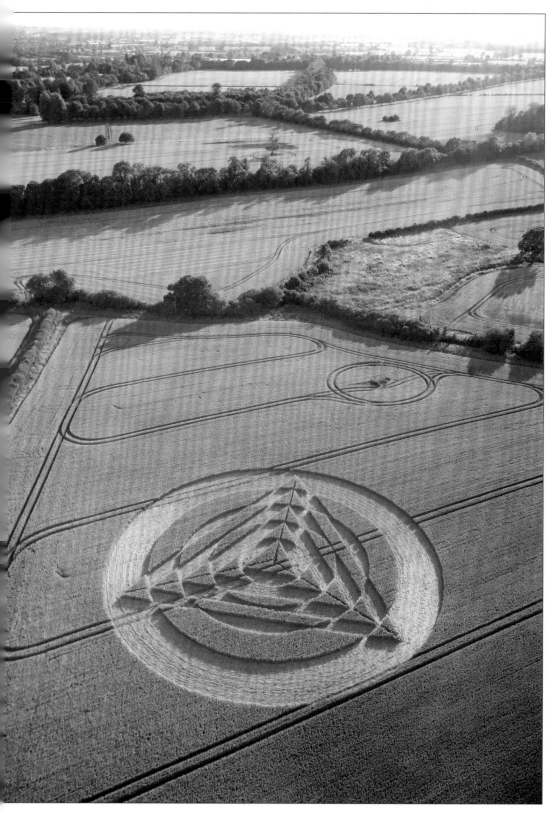

Fig. 1.13. Tetbury Lane, near Charlton, Wiltshire, July 8, 2014.

environment is far less known and still little accepted. The primary reason for this is that even mainstream practitioners are totally unaware of the two domains of science.

However, the concept of mind and matter (see Descartes) is well documented in ancient philosophy.

The modern view is that mind only exists in the brain; whereas a more appropriate description is that we are like sponges in the ocean. Mind permeates the body with measurable frequencies from around the Earth's Schumann frequency of some 8 Hz to around 20 kHz. Analysis of these frequencies using the latest EEG equipment will enable correlations to be made between the embedded frequencies due to, say, Parkinson's disease and how ambient crop circle frequencies can retune the brain, at least on a temporary basis, as currently understood.

The latest radionics equipment, now entering the European market, will not only be able to detect frequency misalignment problems but will be able to retune the appropriate mistuned body functions. This will lead us to a further understanding of the crop circle element. This is the future of medicine. The crop circle scenario is leading the way.

2

"ONENESS" AND COSMIC CONSCIOUSNESS

How can you prove whether at this moment we are sleeping, and all our thoughts are a dream; or whether we are awake, and talking to one another in the waking state?

PLATO (427–347 BCE),

SOME OF THE MOST OUTSTANDING and beautiful reports I have received over the many years are ones where people have experienced sensations of "uplift-ment," peace, Universal Love, and a feeling of "Oneness" with all mankind. So intense have these been at times that the person has struggled to express it in the ordinary Earth-time words we use.

I regret to admit that one of our national failings in Britain is our seem-ing inability to talk to strangers easily. We are naturally reserved. Many are the stories of professionals traveling up to London by train (or elsewhere) to work, sitting in the same carriage with the same occupants for years and still not knowing their names. Our customary method is to hastily bury our heads in the morning or evening newspaper, having bid a general "good morning" or "goodbye," and that's all!

So, as a result, finding that we are actually talking quite happily to strang-ers inside a crop circle is well outside our normal behavior, and it is even more astonishing to actually experience a sense of "Oneness" with the other people present—a remarkable experience indeed for us who are sometimes regarded as being "stuffy" Brits! So what is happening?

Just as we sometimes find that we are on the same wavelength as another person, owing to our frequencies being compatible (a scientific explanation), so when we are inside the circle we have entered a different Consciousness in which all our frequencies have unconsciously gelled together in a unique union of "energy." This feeling of Universal Love and "Oneness" continues for some time after leaving the crop circle.

Often have I been inside a circle and been able to see and hear the traffic roaring by but at the same time have not been a part of it, but "outside" it, having a feeling of being in a different world, safe and secure as though back in the womb, with the two existences acting simultaneously.

Entering the circles, I find that there is a pull and desire to sit and meditate and let myself drift away into other dimensions, other levels of consciousness. In these altered states ideas can often pop into one's head so unexpectedly that one wonders where on Earth they came from! Indeed I believe they do not come from our often rather dense earthly energy states here on Earth but from an exterior energy outside our being. Once when I was sitting quietly meditating, I became aware that I was surrounded in light. It was a strong white light tempered by pale pink, lilac, and orange. The light was constantly moving and I felt happy and peaceful except for pressure round my temples where the white light seemed to be trying to penetrate.

I made my body into a hollow shell and allowed the white light to enter, letting it pass down to all regions, being conscious of its passage as it went. My fingers and toes started to tingle a lot, and my whole body became light, not just in color but also in substance. It seemed as though the light were adjusting the chakras as it passed along.

One has to wonder from whence comes the inspiration for certain musicians to write such glorious and soul-linking music that transports a person into another world. Similarly the same question could be asked of poets, singers, and artists working in other forms of art. Indeed the frequencies involved seem to play a major part in this, and as demonstrated in later chapters in this book, number and music are related, and crop circles are giving off unseen frequencies, influencing our inner beings.

Over the years many groups have attempted to link into the consciousness behind the crop circles in order to manifest a circle of a particular shape, design, or construction—some with extraordinary success.

Perhaps the major outcome of crop circles and Earth Energy effects in general is that the phenomenon is closely linked to human consciousness. It is as if formations appear according to an unpredictable amalgam of human intent!

It is clearly being revealed that the dominant paradigm will in due course be seen to be holistic, implying the connectivity of everything. The interaction of our intent with the Cosmos is already (re)establishing itself as a major factor in our overall understanding of how the Universe functions.

One example was reported by Simon Masters, who sent me this intriguing report.

CROP CIRCLES AND INTENTIONALITY

On Thursday, July 23, 2009, around thirty local people attended a talk by Glenn Broughton, a visiting researcher, tour guide, and expert on the subject of "Crop Circles" at Sheldon village hall, near Dunkerswell.

The following day the crop circle [shown in figures 2.1 and 2.2] was reported.

What follows is an account of the processes that immediately predated and postdated the appearance of the pattern [in figure 2.1] and were connected by group intentionality.

My homework for the event had consisted of a cursory review of internet photography of crop circles. Some of these I had earmarked as "fakes" in the sense that I believed them to be photographic manipulations. Prior to the meeting I had been impressed by the artistic form of the circles, which have developed both in terms of intricacy and sophistication of execution since I last reviewed the phenomenon. Simple circles, such as the one that appeared on the Millerton bypass that kindled my personal interest some fifteen years ago, are not significant news any longer.

During the meeting's Q and A session I asked: "As someone who has visited over 250 crop patterns, what kind of intelligence do you feel lies behind the phenomenon?"

Glenn had suggested that he did not want to give explanations, but described his sense that "[the intelligence is] a playful one, one that enjoys interacting with human minds."

Several of us remarked that we found this comment very interesting.

The scientist in me called on me to find a rational and simple explanation for the patterns I see. Employing Occam's Razor I conclude the creators have to be a group of [human] land artists, some of whom are involved in the occult studies of divine proportion and sacred geometry and who have a remarkable talent for evading detection during the creation of their art.

Glen however had earlier described an "experiment" he had conducted with another group, in which the individuals present had, effectively, "asked the circle creators to produce a circle for them." He reported that— remarkably, and as if on cue—the next significant pattern to be reported had held, for him, a personal and a numerical connection with his experiment. Although inelegant, the pattern reported contained the same number of circles as minds engaged with the experiment.

My response was to encourage Glenn to continue to conduct such experiments in a "scientific" manner, but given that we all appeared to share Glenn's "sense of the playful," could we play now? I cannot remember precisely but I asked, "Is everyone here up for a group meditation, with the intention of asking the Circle Makers to create a work that speaks to us as a group?" The hall was hastily cleared of chairs, and twenty-five people held hands and were taken through a guided thought process by Glenn's wife, Cameron.

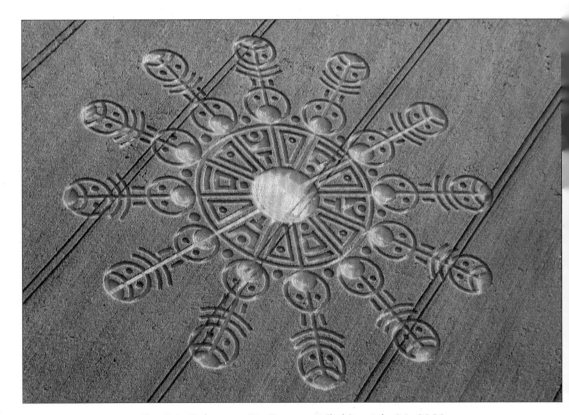

Fig. 2.1. Ogbourne St. George, Wiltshire, July 24, 2009.

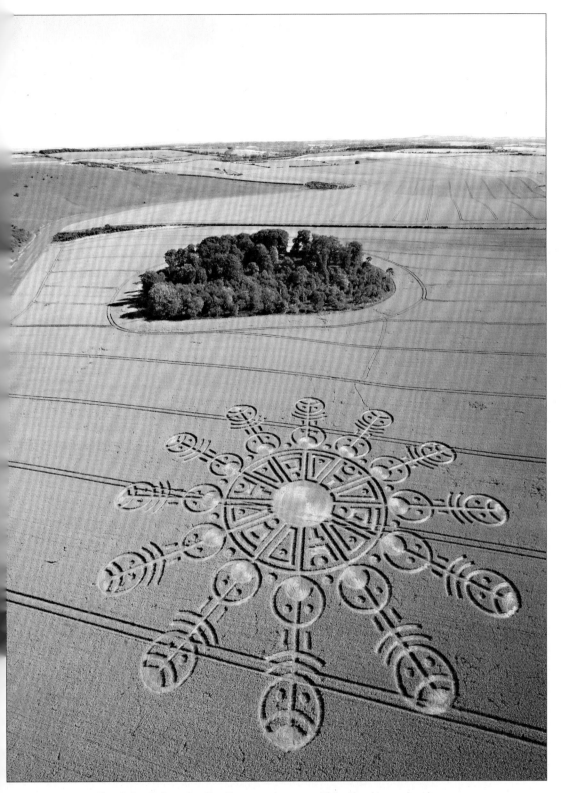

Fig. 2.2. Ogbourne St. George shown within the larger landscape,
Wiltshire, July 24, 2009.

Those unwilling to participate were unobtrusive observers or had left the hall by this stage, and in a ten-minute exercise that was not without mirth and laughter, the group focused their intent on building "our" crop circle pattern.

There was no mention of specificity of timing or pattern. I remember being surprised that, as well as counting the participants (I was number 8 and Sarah 9), Glenn showed some interest in the fact that sixteen females and nine males took part. My personal state was one of "contentment" and "nonattachment to outcome," and I was not cognizant of my gender during the meditation.

As mentioned above, the following day a formation was reported. Since reading the report on Saturday the twenty-sixth, my mind has been periodically intensely reflective on the process and finding some form of explanation or meaning for what has happened. I have an interest in practical magic, but it is not every day I attempt a collaborative manifestation or demonstration of this nature.

Some specific aspects of "connectedness" or cause-and-effect phenomena may be worth mentioning.

1. In later discussion, it emerged that Glenn had the intention of doing a guided meditation but was reluctant to initiate such an exercise with an unfamiliar group. It would seem that my spontaneous suggestion facilitated his intent. Furthermore I noted my ego—my reaction to this—and was pleasantly surprised to find "I" felt comfortable with my contribution to the group process.

2. The pattern consists of 12 large and 12 small circles, plus a central circle, making 25 circles in all. The pattern has the layout of a clock face and therefore can be interpreted as depicting an analogue device for measuring time. It also has the gross symmetry of a snowflake. Closer examination reveals threefold rotational symmetry.

3. We can note that 9 (males) + 16 (females) = 25 (circles) = 12 + 12 + 1, but also that $3^2+4^2=5^2$. That is to say the numbers of males and females associated with the creative process have a relation to a right angled triangle of sides 3, 4, and 5 units in length, and of course that the formation is one solution to the Dionysian polynomial: $x^2 + y^2 = z^2$.

4. Our group met near Dunkerswell, which is one of three aerodrome fields built principally by the Americans during World War II on the Blackdown Hills. The others are at Smeatharpe and Tricky Warren (Culmhead). The pattern appeared at Smeathe's Plantation near Ogbourne Down Gallop, Wiltshire.

My position oscillates between "belief" that we had some cause-and-effect relationship to this particular circle, and "rejection" that the whole thing is coincidence. The following explanations (or cause-and-effect models) exist:

- "Our" circle does not exist; it is a Photoshop hoax.
- "Our" circle exists, but the numerical coincidence is insignificant and there is no cause-and-effect (or synchronicity) relationship between what took place at Sheldon and the Smeathe's Plantation crop circle.
- "Our" circle exists, but there was direct human-to-human communication between one or more people present at Sheldon village hall and the "artist" behind "our" circle.
- These explanations are not mutually exclusive.

My coauthor James Lyons said, "So, in conclusion, the phenomenon is not explained and I suggest that further work is required."

Is there indeed a consciousness inherent in the crop circle that links itself to the human mind/body or vice versa? To me the answer is a resounding yes, as shown by this story.

Researcher Marvin Naylor reported,

When I was there in the Cheesefoot Head circle, two women turned up. One in her seventies, the other late forties, I think. They said they didn't know exactly where the formation was but sensed it—they could "feel" it in their stomachs—as they got nearer in the car. They said it was quite common for them to get that feeling, especially with fresh formations, and especially the younger one. I said they should contact you and tell you. (I said I'd tell you, anyway.) So you might hear from them.

THE OPEN DOOR

A final strange event occurred this past summer of 2018. I met Sue Dury at an airfield as she was waiting to fly after one of my crop circle tours. This is a very popular optional extra of the tour. Flying over the crop circles and the surrounding ancient sites, such as the wonderful Avebury stone complex and Silbury Hill, adds to the magic of the whole day as we soar over

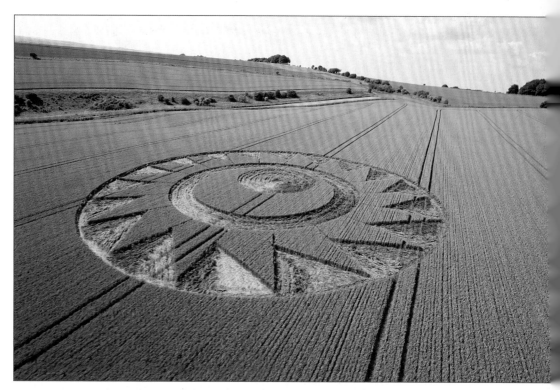

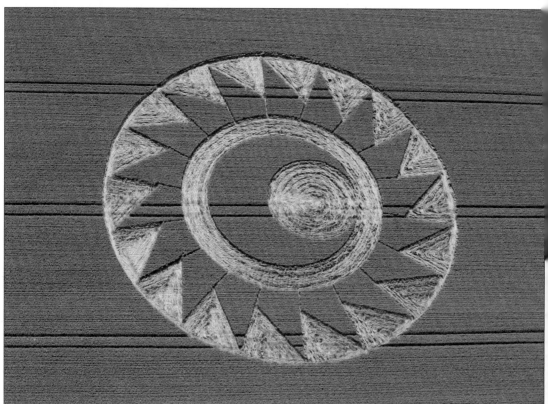

Figs. 2.3 and 2.4. Cheesefoot Head, near Winchester, Hampshire, June 17, 2017.

the sacred landscape of our ancestors seeing it in all its glory below.

Her son Josh was with her, and he too had had a strange experience, but it is hers I am going to tell you about due to its extraordinary uniqueness.

When Josh and I went to visit a Crop Circle Formation at Yarnbury Castle on the 25th of June, we sat down inside the circle. After discussing white balls of light, Josh told me that if you ask the crop circle makers for a certain design they would make it for you. I would like to think that I am a very down-to-earth person but thought I would give it a go.

I said out loud, "Crop circle makers if you really exist then please can you make me a design of a door or window?" (I was thinking of moving house at the time.) This design was really off the wall as normally the designs are of stars or flowers.

I said, "If you make this for me then I will believe in you."

Lo and Behold, a month later, a crop circle formation was reported at Fovant and guess what it was of? A Door!!!

I couldn't believe it as it was such a strange design to ask for. Nobody could have overheard our conversation. There was nobody else there! I felt this one was made for me.

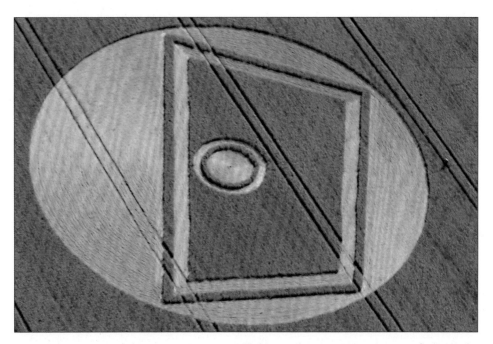

Fig. 2.5. Gurston Ashes, near Fovant, Wiltshire, July 23, 2018, circa 90 ft (27.5m) diameter. Wheat circle containing a rectangular door.

I have to believe in the crop circle makers now as they did what I asked for.

Josh asked me what connection I had with Fovant. The only connection I had with Fovant was that I took my mother to see the white chalk badges many years ago now. She has since passed but it makes you wonder if there is a spiritual connection. Was it my mother's way of contacting me? I have no answer for this.

The circle was lying hidden above the White Chalk Military Badges carved into the hillside above Fovant and was hard to find. Yet again we have this connection with the Universal Conscious Mind in all its teasing and Puckish ways.

What is this telling us, I wonder? As with many crop circles, it is open to multiple interpretations that may be whispering different words to both you and me. Bizarre and indeed trite as the crop circle may seem at first glance, when one looks into this image more deeply, one starts to question what an opening door could be saying to us? What does it mean?

An open door, may be giving us the opportunity of "opening" us to a new direction in life, new opportunities, accessing new dimensions, or raising us to

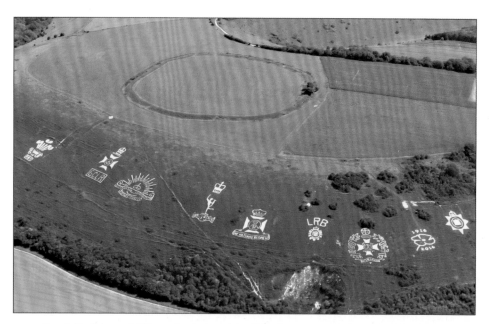

Fig. 2.6. Fovant Military Badges with Chiselbury Megalithic Hill Fort in the background. The badges L to R: 1. Royal Wiltshire Yeomanry. 2. 6th City of London) Battalion, London Regiment (City of London Rifles). 3. Australian Commonwealth Military Forces. 4. Royal Corps of Signals. 5. Wiltshire Regiment. 6. 5th (City of London Battalion), London Regiment (London Rifle Brigade). 7. 8th (City of London) Battalion, London Regiment (Post Office Rifles) 8. Devonshire Regiment.

other levels of consciousness. Whatever the answer, I see it as quite one of the most important and inspirational circles of 2018.

I believe that we are all part of the Universal Consciousness, which is multidimensional and multi-interactional. This being so, we have to take on board the awesome fact that in this we are indeed all part of each other.

COMMENTS BY JAMES LYONS

Hitherto the topic of conscious connection to crop formations and Earth Energy effects in general has been virtually unknown territory in mainstream science. However, many recent long-range conscious effects, ranging from Transcendental Meditation to quantum entanglement have been thoroughly investigated. These studies indicate that "intent" is a key part of cosmic processes.

One very recent theory to emerge in the last decade is Global Scaling Theory. This is based on the concept that the Universe is structured on the basis of standing cosmic waves in logarithmic space. This technical term is in principle similar to the way that harmonic structures are an integral part of music.

If objects have been physically linked then separated, they remain consciously connected—a key example being the case of identical twins. Alternatively, focusing mentally on any scene, however distant, also establishes a link between the person creating intent and the object of visualization. It is currently being suggested that the standing wave resembles a vortex filament, something well known in physics, particularly Cosmology.

Since by definition a standing wave does not propagate, its nodes are the key elements of the wave, which are coherently linked. This means that information available at either node is instantaneously available at the other. This process is essentially a holographic scenario.

The research organization* undertaking this work has used the technique to transmit messages even from Europe to Australia by tapping directly into this universal energy field! The process is showing remarkable similarities to the nonlocal conscious effects observed in the crop circle phenomenon.

Patterns of Intent from one or more meditators can collectively create orbs, which are capable of coherently forming and manifesting patterns closely based on the combined thought processes of the participants.

---

*See *Global Scaling* by Andreas Beutel (Munich: FQL Publishers, 2008).

3

DOWSING IN CROP CIRCLES AND LABYRINTHS

No man can reveal to you aught but that which already lies half asleep in the dawning of your knowledge. For the vision of one man lends not its wings to another man.

THE PROPHET BY KAHLIL GIBRAN (1883–1931)

I ALWAYS ORGANIZE AN ANNUAL CROP CIRCLE scientific research day (see chapter 8), and scientist and dowser Bob Sephton was one of my regular attendees for many years until his health prevented him from coming. In 2014 he wrote telling me that

> my bladder cancer has returned so I am now having chemo from time to time during the next few weeks. I decided to summarize all my defects/problems on a list and see what can be done. Cancer, left ankle "shattered" (some years ago), left eyesight not too good, balance is terrible, both knees stiff, kidneys not too good, to name a few. I am eighty-six in a few weeks' time but NOT yet ready to "bow out."
>
> I dowsed that I could do something about all this. Chemicals—No, Homeopathic—Yes. But I don't have all of them. "Yes you do! You are looking at photographs from your Crop Circles Calendar." . . . In front of me was a scrap book in which each year I stick in photographs from your Crop Circles Calendar.
>
> I dowsed which Crop Circle would be appropriate for a specific problem.

Holding his pendulum over the appropriate circle for each ailment, it would start spinning and stop when the treatment was completed.

So make of this what you will. It is having an effect; some results have worked quicker than others. The European Union is trying to make a rule that only doctors can prescribe homeopathic treatments, which means that they will not. So do your own by dowsing for the selected image; place a hand over the appropriate photograph and use your pendulum to tell you when one has had enough; it is as simple as that. Check from time to time to see if one has to change the photo for the problem.

I am a migraine sufferer and had been enduring terrible headaches for almost two weeks, which my normal medicine and powders were doing nothing to relieve. So when I received Bob Sephton's email I thought—why not give it a try?

Getting out several of my old calendars and sitting comfortably in a chair, I started dowsing image after image . . . nothing . . . nothing . . . then suddenly my pendulum went wild over the beautifully harmonious 2013 Hackpen formation. Amazed, I got a larger overhead image of the circle and stared at it. Horrors, it was all jagged and sharp and really unpleasant. Could I bear to go on looking? My pendulum never lies to me, so I persevered and got more and more fascinated as the circle started to change shape before my eyes. It evolved into 3-D patterns! How long I watched all this happening I really don't know, but suddenly I realized that I no longer had a migraine! It had gone completely.

I now keep a photograph of this formation in my bag alongside the powders as a fallback, as it is not always possible to find a place to sit and stare at a photograph!

A BIRTHDAY PRESENT

Not long after this experience I was giving a talk at the lovely Glastonbury Symposium and, as always, I finish with a musical slide show of crop circle images from over the years. This is always popular—an emotional release into other wonderful levels of consciousness. I was sent a lovely, heartwarming report by one of the viewers.

Thank you for your wonderful presentation on crop circles at the Glastonbury Symposium, and for taking the time to search for the crop

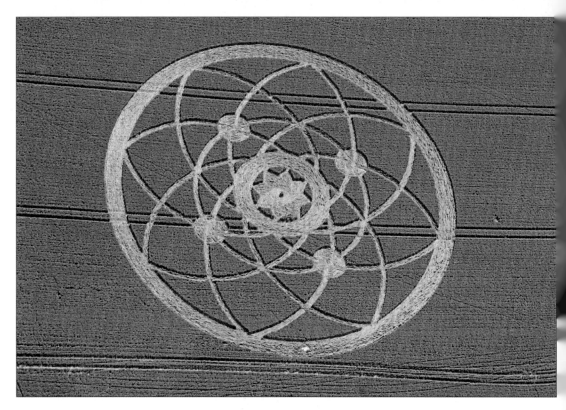

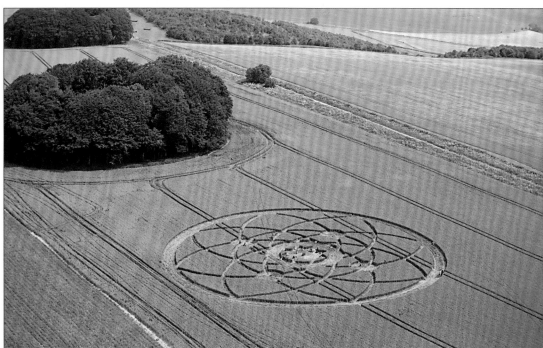

Figs. 3.1 and 3.2. Two views of the Hackpen Hill formation, near Broad Hinton, Wiltshire, reported July 15, 2013. A circle containing an eightfold floral pattern with a central octagon surrounded by a flattened ring approximately 80 feet in diameter in wheat.

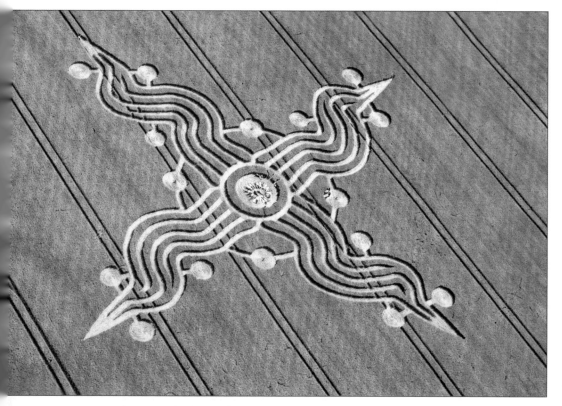

Fig. 3.3. West Woods, Lockeridge, Wiltshire, July 17, 2008.

circle that created my episode of intense emotion, which combined feelings of "love, release, knowing, and meaning."

It wasn't until your presentation on July 27 (my fifty-first birthday!) that I realized "my past, my present, and my future" . . . in other words "my purpose" came to being. The first three crop circles (they were different views of the same circle) that you showed in your "sight and sound" presentation hit me so powerfully that I wasn't able to breathe; I had an intense release of emotion . . . feelings of "love/release/knowing/meaning." . . . I had palpitations in a point above my heart, which I have now learned is the "Thymus Chakra."

As we travel further into the different areas of healing we find we are treading an unlikely and unexpected path. How could it be that labyrinths, dowsing, and healing are part of the same interwoven fabric?

It is only as we continue our journey of exploration that we find that certain threads connect all three.

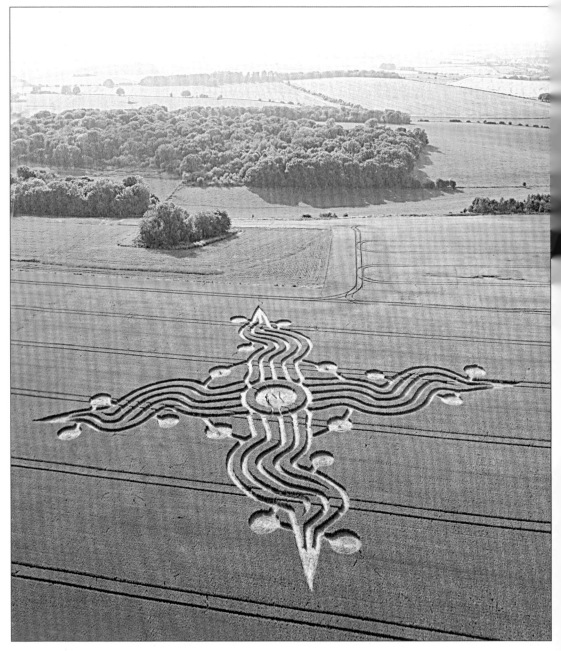

Fig. 3.4. West Woods, Lockeridge, Wiltshire, July 17, 2008.

HUNT THE CIRCLE

Many years ago when the crop circles were appearing in great quantities in Hampshire, I had a strange and somewhat uncomfortable experience. Ex–Second World War Burma bomber pilot and renowned dowser David Russell had flown over and seen from the air a crop circle in a field just off the A272 in

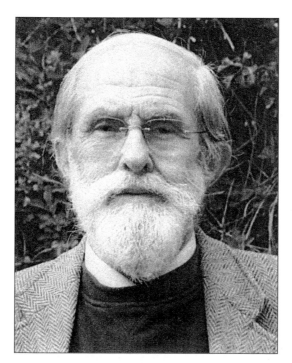

Fig. 3.5. David Russell.

Hampshire near Winchester. Realizing that the circle was on flat ground and would be difficult to find, and while the image was still clear in his mind, he made his way to the field as soon as he landed and managed to find it.

David had found some very interesting dowsing patterns and had asked me to see what I could detect with my pendulum. Needless to say, I never did find it, so it seemed a heaven-sent opportunity when some four or five weeks later, on a soaking wet day, we went on an expedition to try and locate it together with Hamish Miller (who discovered the Michael and Mary ley lines and is author of *The Sun and the Serpent*) and David's wife, Barbara.

We made our way to the field. There was a path running the length of the field down one side. It soon became clear to us that we were going to have difficulty locating the circle for as far as our eyes could reach was an endless sea of barley and no vantage point from which to see into the crop.

I realized that I had left my pendulum in the car parked some distance away from the field, and I had not even brought my dowsing rods either. Drat and double drat! As we were walking down the path suddenly I felt a tight band around my head. "Stop," I called to David, who had gone ahead. "The circle is here," I said, pointing into the field. David felt sure it was further on but as the band around my head seemed to be tightening still more, he obligingly went into the field but went off at an angle and soon was lost to sight in the waves of pale golden stalks of barley. In despair I borrowed Barbara's dowsing rods and asked them to indicate where the circle was. They pointed straight into the field from where we were standing, and I entered where David had, but instead of going off at an oblique angle, I followed the rods down the tramline at 90 degrees to the path. It seemed as though we were walking forever, and I started to doubt my dowsing ability—however, some 70 or 80 yards later I suddenly saw the circle literally two steps in front of me. It was a beautiful double ringer, which clearly had had few if any other visitors apart from David and now us. The moment I stepped into it an extraordinary thing happened; the band of steel was completely lifted from my poor aching head. What a relief!

I have spoken to several people since that experience, and I am told that it is a well-known fact that we may use our bodies as dowsing instruments. However since that day, I always make a point of trying to remember to bring my rods in order to locate circles in this way, as so many of them are not visible from the ground. I am sure most dowsers do the same. Bands of steel do not appeal to me, so I am always careful to make sure I have my rods or pendulum with me, I even used my handbag once, but I suppose it is a useful means if all else fails! I have always suffered from a notoriously poor bump of location (sense of direction) but ever since that wet and soggy day, it has improved quite dramatically. Maybe something was unblocked as a result of our expedition!

So many things seem to happen by chance and yet, I ask myself, are they really just "by chance" or are they whisperings which we can either listen to or ignore?

There are many dowsers among my scientific research group who, in addition to being scientists, are in the process of trying to put dowsing on a scientific basis and indeed are close to establishing this.

LONG-DISTANCE COMMUNICATION?

Hugo Jenks (looking like a man from outer space) was busy with his program.

> The angle of my electronic L rod is measured by an angle sensor fitted in the rod handle and plotted on the image as a grey shade. The GPS lat/long position is updated once per second, and so each dot represents one second of measurement at that position.
>
> When the rod is straight ahead it gives a mid-grey dot, when 90 degrees

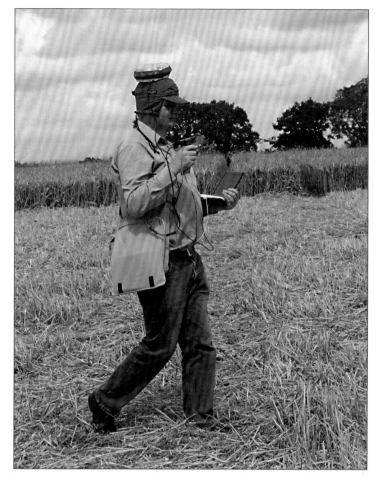

Fig. 3.6. Hugo Jenks during a scientific research day
at Forest Hill, Wiltshire, on July 16, 2014.

or more right it is white, 90 degrees or more left it is black with shades of
grey in between.

I was simply asking to be shown the strength of the energy at the point
where I was walking.

Ideally I would have made my tracks closer together, but I was aware that
there may be limited time. It was quite a large area; to cover it in fine detail
would take several hours.

It is also hard work to maintain focus. For example at about the three
o'clock position there is a large area of consistent white indicated about
20 meters long and 8 meters wide. However, you will see a kink in my path,
and no indicated energy. My focus went from dowsing to avoiding some people

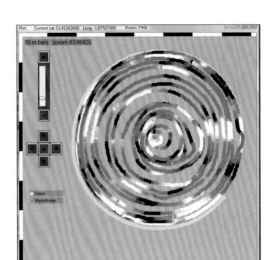

Fig. 3.7. Hugo Jenks's GPS results.

standing there. So the indications in that kink section are to be ignored.

I have a button on the handle. When pressed the dot is shown as yellow. I use that to draw the outline of physically visible items, such as hedges or standing stones, in this case the perimeter of the circle.

Note that the indicated GPS position does wander a little. So the yellow outline does not quite meet the point where I started, by about a meter (see fig. 3.7). Not too bad really on this scale, but be aware that consistent measurements of small scales are hard to achieve with the GPS wandering around by +/− a meter or so. Hence some energy lines although straight in reality can appear a bit jagged.

I do feel we need a scientific approach to dowsing. It will take some legwork to get there.

The big advantage of my rod is that the indication is continuously variable, like the volume control on a radio. It has the ability to indicate subtle features if repeated on successive tracks. The eye can pick out the feature afterward even if you did not notice a particularly strong response at the time. Usually those who use flags have to make a decision at the time of dowsing whether to place the flag or not. It is like the on-off button on a radio. You have to listen to it full blast or not at all. Placing the flag also forces you to switch your mental mode from being receptive to being decisive and back. With my system, provided you can maintain focus, you can remain continuously in the receptive mode.

FINDING THE WAY

So how do labyrinths fit into this equation? The crop circle phenomenon takes me all over the world giving talks—to places I would never have the opportunity to visit otherwise. One of these was to lecture at the Labyrinth Society's annual conference in Taos, New Mexico, in the autumn of 2014. Was it by chance that two wonderful crop circle labyrinths had appeared as heralds in the fields in Wiltshire that very summer? After giving my lecture I was given an introduction to labyrinth designer and builder Marty Cain.

In June of 1994, about twelve people came to a workshop I gave in conjunction with an art project called "Art in Nature" sponsored by the New Art Center in Newton, Massachusetts, and the National Endowment for the Arts. I taught them all to dowse. We each walked my temporary labyrinth marked with white turkey feathers and used our new skill to find our way into the

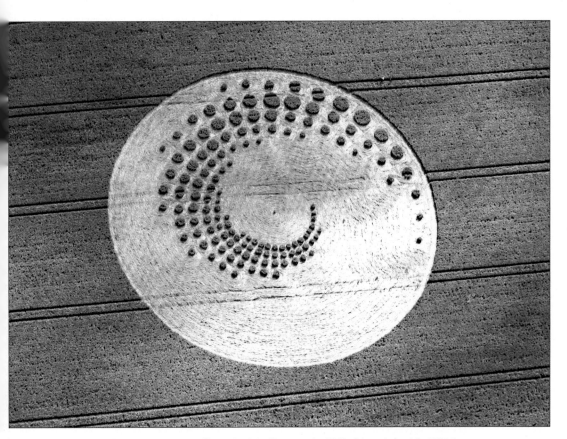

Fig. 3.8. Forest Hill, near Marlborough, Wiltshire, July 16, 2014.

park and locate sacred spots of our own. At the end of the day one woman shared that she had once been attacked in the woods and had not gone near a forest in years. This day she overcame her fear and followed her dowsing rods deep into the woods. She was elated with this new freedom and gave credit to walking the labyrinth. Others reported insights and told me of being cleared from mental blocks. There was an overall sense of well-being, wonder, and fun.

Another Massachusetts art project found me working with special-education students at Somerville High School. The Somerville Arts Council commissioned me to work with them to build a community labyrinth at the Somerville Growing Center, a block down Vinal Street from the high school. I showed the students slides of ancient sites, taught the teens to dowse, and to draw the labyrinth. We worked together using donated bricks imbedded in the new turf so there would be a minimum of maintenance and allow for the varied use of the space. The students all had special needs that kept them from taking regular classes. One boy, I'll call him Jim, had never spoken a full sentence in his life.

We walked down to the garden center, dowsed the form, and marked it with blue surveyors' flags and tape. Together we created a blessing, walked in procession through the labyrinth, and then headed back up the hill for lunch in the school cafeteria. That afternoon we were to return to start cutting the turf and placing the bricks to mark the paths. Jim called to his teacher saying, "I wish I could come back after lunch but I have health class." Everybody stopped in their tracks. Even Jim was shocked. After lunch Jim and the whole health class came to the garden center to walk the labyrinth.

The next day Jim would not walk the labyrinth. I asked why. "Lost," he said. "Lost!" Finally he managed to have me understand that his family relied on the income the state provided for his disability and that he had never been taught enough to keep up with normal students and would be lost. "Lost!" He said. Not in the labyrinth but in his life. I suggested that he continue to work on the project and in two years when he was to grad-uate and his obligation to his family was fulfilled, he return to walk the labyrinth. He could start his education newly, fully able to express himself. We embraced, both with tears in our eyes. Later the staff of the growing center said he was always there, working to keep the labyrinth perfect. What happened to this boy in the labyrinth? I do not know, but I was more deter-mined than ever to understand the power of walking a labyrinth.

In the early nineties I had teamed up with Dr. Wayne London of Brattleboro, Vermont, to study the effects of using sacred space to heal diseases. During a workshop in Putney, Vermont, a seventy-two-year-old gentleman, who had been suffering with Parkinson's disease for fifteen years, shuffled slowly into the center of a small temporary labyrinth that I had dowsed and marked with mounds of hay and surveyors flags. When he came out he was taking full strides and smiling from ear to ear. All symptoms of his crippling disease had vanished. I chanced to meet him four months later and noticed that his symptoms were returning. When I offered to build a labyrinth at his home in Virginia he and his wife refused. That was hard for me to understand.

Collaborating again with Wayne London when giving a lecture, this time in Craftsbury, Vermont, people reported being able to see more clearly and richly, with a sense of both more depth and brighter colors. In two other cases their sense of smell was enhanced.

Early one morning a client called me from Georgia to report that a blind priest with Parkinson's disease had just walked her labyrinth supported by his wife. They slowly made their way to the center but, as they were on their way out, he was walking freely and simply holding her hand. Two days later, the couple returned and when the labyrinth owner saw the man walking briskly by himself she ran to the entrance to meet him as he ended his walk. He told her that he was able to go alone because when he had come to the entrance, two gnomes were there to lead him along the paths.

These reports are of people who walked the labyrinth just once or twice. I know of little that has been done to document what happens when labyrinths are walked every day over a long period of time.

So how do we explain how or why this "labyrinth effect" is happening? I think we must refer to Pythagoras: "If we accept that numbers and music are related and labyrinths are constructed not just in geometric forms but in such patterns that give off special frequencies, then the mystery starts to unravel."

THE HEALING ROOM

I believe that so much of this work is all about "frequencies." We are electrical beings interacting with other invisible electrical frequencies. A friend of mine has a special healing room, and she explains that color, as a tool for healing and spiritual development, has been used over many periods of time. Many years ago she worked with an amazing medium who designed a color wheel and she has been using it in her healing room for over thirty years. It is an electrical machine that simply consists of two discs overlaid with colored gels that are arranged in a specific formula. When the machine is switched on, the discs rotate and through the use of a halogen bulb the color is beamed through a projector and reflects onto the wall. This allows a person to come and sit in this energy field and the color is absorbed through the aura and has an effect on the physical condition. She has witnessed a change in a Parkinson's sufferer who came into the room unable to control extensive shaking and who then became perfectly still and relaxed.

She never consciously chooses a specific color for anyone. She prepares the room and allows the wheel to stop randomly, always bearing in mind her connection with the spirit world and the power that can be invoked for that particular person. Everyone is different, and it depends on the soul itself as to whether it is time for a condition to be removed or whether there is still more to be learned from it.

She further explains that we have to understand that the soul is a vehicle of light expressing itself through the color spectrum according to the changing thought pattern. "As we think, so it is." Therefore, the aura surrounding the physical body is an electrical force field continually feeding the individual and changing the molecular and chemical structure. This has a great influence on the health of the human being.

COMMENTS BY JAMES LYONS

Dowsing has been used by our forefathers to detect the flowing spiraling telluric currents in the earth. These form a grid network north-south and east-west. At crossover points we find spiderweb-like patterns. All ancient sites up to the time of medieval churches are constructed on so-termed Earth acupuncture points. These points are key to where crop circles occur. Since our conscious interaction with all Earth Energies depends on receiving ambient energy structure, we simply ask appropriate questions to analyze crop circle structures.

So with dowsing we find the underlying telluric "graph paper" on which crop circles form. This allows us to record in great detail the pattern's fundamental geometries, which were first discovered and recorded by the ancient Greeks. This is all called sacred geometry. We analyze the underground energy patterns almost always focusing on water sources. These are the source of energy, which rises in bubble rings from below, creating crop patterns as the crop is flattened. Dowsing can be used to measure the relevant energy distribution across a formation.

The information one can extract from crop circles is very diverse. First, it explains how human consciousness is but one element in dissecting how Nature functions in general. We are involved in an interchange of dynamically evolving ideas. It clearly shows that we ourselves are immersed in this self-organizing field—we hold a conversation. Healing is but one aspect of this dialogue.

Using aerial photos, it is also possible to measure from the geometry the key harmonic features of a formation. These are almost without exception based on the harmonics of the diatonic scale, first defined by Pythagoras. It is usually possible using dowsing to establish how a pattern was laid down.

If, say, a pattern is based on a series of circles, then a procedure analogous to embroidery is involved, with a column of energy spiraling up through the ground thus creating a localized circle, then descending back to Earth reemerging in another location. In this way sequences of circles appear to create an overall composite pattern. It is often the case that dowsing is used on aerial photos to work out the creation mechanism.

What is unique about crop circles is the apparent intelligence behind some patterns. This author on several occasions has encountered formations in the field that are closely aligned with a priori computer images hypothesized some time earlier. This effect clearly demonstrates that the conscious link is key to the process.

Dowsing is the modern word to describe how not only humans but also all animals, birds, and fishes interact with the all-pervading cosmic energy. The Ancients call this the *Aether,* while modern science calls it either the "quantum vacuum" or the "zero-point energy field." It is the fount of all knowledge (the ancient Akashic Records). It acts as an all-knowing library like the modern internet, which one can interrogate. Time and distance are of no relevance.

This is why the phenomenon so attracts those people of spiritual backgrounds. While we use dowsing to measure the energy absorbed by the crops, we still struggle to fully determine the obvious intelligence behind the phenomenon. This remains a work in progress.

4

FREQUENCIES
AND LUMINOSITIES

As we acquire knowledge, things do not become more comprehensible, but more mysterious.

ALBERT SCHWEITZER (1875–1965)

WHAT IS IT THAT IS AFFECTING us when we go into crop circles?

As already mentioned in the book, we appear to be entering a "sphere of influence" that has a profound effect on certain people. Could a change in frequency be the case?

All the reports given below are in connection with crop circles, but just as with other crop circle effects these same effects and phenomena have been recorded in lesser number in and around ancient stone circles. It would appear that there is an ambient electrical field connecting the electrical field of the stones and the residual electromagnetic field of the crop circle force that interacts in a glorious marriage with the existing ambient field of certain energetic spots in the landscape. These fields were understood by our ancient ancestors, whose knowledge of the stars, the seasons, and the natural world leaves us, in our manic world of technology, struggling to catch up with them. We are only just now starting to relearn and appreciate this wisdom.

We will begin our investigation with oral reports. Just as I have experienced many of the previous effects having visited hundreds of circles, so this one is of particular interest.

I CAN'T GET THAT
TASTE OUT OF MY MOUTH

On certain occasions when entering a formation, I get this strange metallic taste in my mouth that is so pervasive I cannot get rid of it by spitting or drinking or by any other means. I only ever experience this when in these circumstances, never at any other time. Other people have also experienced this taste, and Debbie Benstead considers it her litmus test as to the genuineness of a formation. Since discussing this taste in talks, I have been amazed by the number of people who have also experienced this sensation. Shelly Keel has also reported a "metallic/acid taste in my mouth." Shelly has no metal, amalgam, or gold fillings in her mouth.

The most interesting story of all came from a woman who approached me after my talk at the 1995 CCCS Conference in Andover. "I have that taste in my mouth *now*," she announced, "and I am not in a crop circle, *but* I am a diet-maintained diabetic!" She went on to tell me that whenever her protein ketones rise to a certain level she experiences this "taste" and has to get something to eat quickly in order to correct this situation. In other words this is her warning signal that her blood-sugar level is dropping dramatically, and she must do something about it.

What are ketones? They are organic compounds that contain a carbonyl group (an oxygen atom doubly bonded to a carbon atom) bonded to two other organic groups. The blood ketone level in humans normally increases in response to starvation, diabetes mellitus, or a high-fat, low-carbohydrate diet. Dietary changes and, in diabetes, the administration of insulin usually correct the condition.

On another occasion after I had given a talk at Chevy Chase, Maryland, during a lecture tour of the States and Canada, Larry Arnold, who has spent twenty-three years researching spontaneous human combustion,* approached me in great excitement to tell me that whereas few people survive spontaneous human combustion, he had an account of such a person, a woman who, when interviewed after the terrible event, reported experiencing the same metallic taste.

Clearly it is of electrochemical origin and can occur when an electrical field of specific frequency and amplitude triggers gustatory (sense of taste) receptors.

---

*See *Ablaze! The Mysterious Fires of Spontaneous Human Combustions* by Larry E. Arnold (New York: M. Evans, 1995; ISBN: 0-87131-789-3).

SPONTANEOUS COMBUSTION

A recent theory suggests that spontaneous combustion may be due to chronic Candidiasis in which an excess amount of internal alcohol, resulting from a yeast infection, floods the bloodstream. If the body attempts to eliminate the alcohol through the skin, this will create a bubble of alcohol, vapor around the body. If the sufferer goes near a candle or cooking flame or lights a cigarette or pipe, the body will spontaneously combust.

Furthermore, Charles Dickens in *Bleak House* described the death of heavy drinker Krook:

> Here is a small burnt patch of flooring; here is the tender from a little bundle of burnt paper, but not so light as usual, seeming to be steeped in something; and here is—is it the cinder of a small charred and broken log of wood sprinkled with white ashes, or is it coal, O Horror, he is here! And this, from which we run away, striking out the light and overturning one another into the street, is all that represents him.

When their bodies touch the fallen crop inside a crop circle, people often experience throbbing, pulsing, or tingling sensations. "I lay down with my palms on the earth and felt strong pulsing from each fingertip."

DASH TO THE DENTIST

A dramatic oral effect was reported by Dr. Patricia Hill. She suffered from long-standing toxicity since experiencing serious food poisoning in 1984, resulting in autoimmunity, neurological and organ damage, and sensitivity. She had several gold crowns, one titanium implant, and one amalgam filling. She told me,

> I have a strong and peculiar reaction on electrical and electronic devices. Sometimes I have reversed the polarity of such devices, causing them to malfunction or even melt down. I set off alarms, open garage doors, blow up lights, and so forth, and have been studied because of it.

Her story continued:

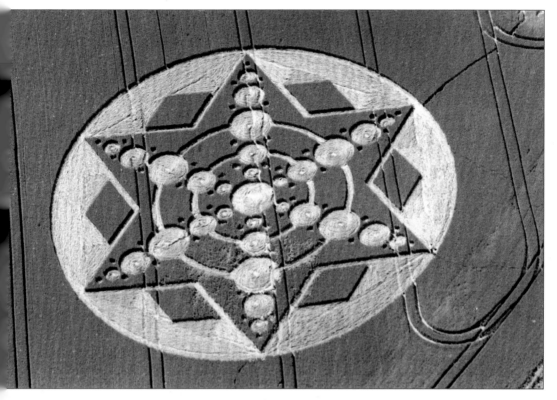

Fig. 4.1. Devil's Den, Clatford, Wiltshire, July 19, 1999.

When friends arrived August 2, 1999, I took them to all the crop circles (starting with Devil's Den), and one of those people, Michelle Rose, and I developed a strange pain in our teeth when we went into the Devil's Den formation. She was so miserable that she was ready to "charter the Concorde" to go home!

Whilst visiting the next formation at Cherhill, blood started gushing from my gums. We both used clove oil, and so forth, to no avail, and she decided to go to a dentist and have a root canal, while I decided to wait until I got home. Due to the pain, neither of us could chew, so we had to eat soft food.

My pain developed into a large abscess between two teeth—a gold crown and another crown—above which is a titanium implant that had broken, exposing the inner core. I had horrible pain going up into my head on the left side, into the back of my head, down my neck, under my chin, into my shoulders, and to my heart.

I used my detox homeopathic on the large swelling and it ruptured, filling my mouth with horrible yellow pus streaked with white. I also used Rescue Remedy, which seemed to help, but I was worried about septicemia, so I went to a doctor and asked for erythromycin.

When I got home I went to my homeopath who was delighted to hear that I had "detoxed" my liver! He pointed out that the place where the abscess had been was a liver point, and all of the places where I had felt extreme pain were also liver points, which had been the cause of my migraine headaches on that side.

My gum and tooth are now fine with no root canal surgery! My headache is also gone!

THE NOISE SEEMED TO BE GETTING LOUDER

Many are the people who have described hearing unusual noises when approaching or being inside crop circles. Indeed several people have developed tinnitus, which they connect directly with their involvement with the circles. The continuous ringing in their ears is an unpleasant sensation.

One report mentions:

I was trying to write down how I was feeling but I could not get my mind to work with my hand so there was a lot of scribbling out along with unprintable language. The noise in my right ear was so loud I was shouting to Colin Andrews, who was with me at the time, telling him what was happening. He was having similar problems.

By moving toward the edge of the formation it seemed to get quieter the closer I got to the edge.

I suffer from tinnitus in my right ear and have done since an experience in a crop circle in 1990, but since I have been in the circle today, the tinnitus has become so loud, I have a job to hear noise from my right ear.

A woman entered another formation and was sitting quietly when she heard a crackling noise in the crop that seemed to be getting louder as it approached her. A couple joined her, and the noise stopped abruptly.

It could be that the stimulation of the hypothalamus is the reason for many of these reports. The cilia in the ear get activated, kicking the neurons in the system into action.

Not all audio effects are negative: a woman member of a Yorkshire group visiting a crop circle below the ancient hill fort at Clay Hill, Wiltshire, recovered from a partial hearing loss problem.

We need to know what frequencies are involved and in which band (VVLF, ELF, LF, HF, VHF, UHF, Microwave). More research is needed in this area.

What is the cause of tinnitus? We are told that tinnitus is the perception of a sound in the ear or head that isn't produced by an outside source. There are many different conditions that can produce tinnitus, and sometimes it can occur for no known reason.

Neuroscience tells us that both sides of the brain are involved in hearing and sound. There is a complex system whereby communication from one ear on one side of the head passes information to identical centers on both sides of the brain. Several parts of the brain are involved in decoding and processing sounds—the brain stem, the midbrain, and the thalamus, and then the temporal lobe of the cerebrum.

PULSING TINY LIGHTS SHAPED LIKE A DOUGHNUT

Lights or luminosities are often associated with crop formations and are seen as stationary, hovering, or moving over a field where the following morning a crop formation is found.

Many people see little balls of light dancing inside the formation. When people report luminosities not seen by other people, it must be asked: Are they describing visual hallucinations or physical sightings?

This is another area where rigid conclusions cannot be drawn. One report tells of a woman who saw "small glistening vortices, whirling around the flattened [grain] toward the perimeter." Another account stated:

A mass of pulsing tiny lights, shaped like a doughnut or a blood cell. It was about three feet across and just one foot high. It didn't come up to me particularly so I was surprised that no one else seemed to notice it. As I watched I could see red streaks like tiny lightning flashes in the sky above the crop. The shaped light was orangey-white. Then it drifted off and speeded up and zoomed off over the hill.

Later that day in Bristol I could see big bouncing orange balls of light following us, bouncing into people and being "absorbed" or dissipating into them!

The story continues with the principal player Win Keech, an engineer currently working as a computer engineer. He has also worked as a designer at Rolls Royce, and was a pilot in the Royal Air Force for a short time.

He has a great interest in UFOs and approaches the topic from a scientific and objective point of view. In 1991 he witnessed a pale luminous disk above the crop in East Field, Alton Barnes, and the subsequent appearance of a small circle. As the disk traveled slowly across the field it was the size of a small dinner plate before expanding to approximately twenty feet in diameter. It then became stationary, hovering over the crop; the wheat beneath shook, rattled, and fell naturally, taking only about three seconds. The disk then moved away across the field contracting as it did so. Keech went to where he had seen the luminous object and found a small circle of approximately twenty feet in diameter.

A final report: "I saw a BOL (ball of light) thirty feet away from me come out of the crop and float over the heads of wheat briefly for around two to three seconds and then disappear."

Other ocular anomalies have occurred in crop circles, such as Christopher Bean's report in which he experienced a "myopic effect" in 1999. (It had also occurred in 1998 when visiting two other formations.) He describes it thus: "It occurs when looking at yellow/green stalks in a large area of flattened crop, the peripheral vision 'zones out' and you get a 'glare' in your central vision. It usually lasts the duration of the visit to the formation."

He also reports that after his visit to the pictogram and "Serpent" in East Field, Alton Barnes, "I was so clumsy for the next two days, ripping my knees and feet open around the house, covering myself in bruises."

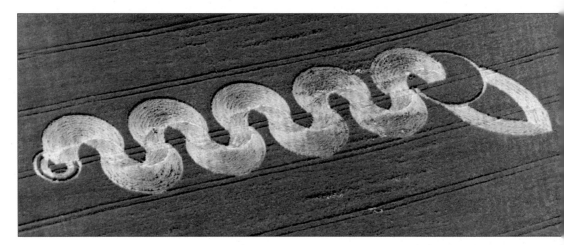

Fig. 4.2. East Field Serpent, Alton Barnes, Wiltshire, June 12, 1999.

A similar report came from a man as he approached the same formation from the direction of the silage pit that lies by the road running from Alton Barnes to Pewsey. As he neared the formation his vision became "whurry" and his whole vision split into two halves with a horizontal line separating the two halves. One section going one way, the other section going the opposite way. His vision was clear in the middle. He does not wear spectacles and has normal vision. He did not see any change in the colors, and it has not happened to him before or since.

Could the cause be due to his normal muscular conversion of the stimulus being spontaneously distorted? The eddy currents in his brain seemed to be affected. We have neurons that run to intraocular muscles. "After some time I noticed that there were colors appearing in my vision (eyes closed); first red and yellow, then turquoise, varying if I moved my eyes up and down."

Seeing various colors internally could be termed as *chromatism,* the hallucinatory perception of colored images, which affect the eddy currents in the brain (neurological sign of brain energies). Pulsed signals, however sourced (visual, acoustic, RF, etc., in very, very low frequency wavelengths), can trigger migraine variant or no headache but other strange symptoms. The person is often "seeing" bright primary colors apparently in the field of view: red, yellow, and turquoise. If projected into the surrounding environment some will interpret the vision as the Virgin Mary (turquoise) or spirits.

Many people have also remarked on a new outer clarity of vision in which the scenery appears as though it is made up of sharply defined "cutouts." A new inner clearness of vision is also often reported, as in the following:

And everything looked enhanced dimensionally. I saw large lines of energy rising from the ground, moving upward, filling the landscape, the horizon, and the sky for hours. The lines were wavy, pulsating, in constant movement. They just kept emanating from the ground.

I kept closing my eyes to try to make it stop—it was like looking at a movie. It was overwhelming—lots of movement. When it got dark that evening, I could see as well as if it was dusk all night. That was one of the things that compelled me to stay outside.

Like I said before, I do see energy but I have not seen anything of that magnitude again. It was like being in a vision, aware of two realities. Things didn't look as they had before. I had fear around this—wondering how long this would last and not really knowing what was happening to me—I felt like I couldn't handle it. When I was able to be briefly still in what I was seeing and observe it, I had an overwhelming feeling of vastness, wonder, and love—like things I had known deep within about other states of consciousness and dimensions were real.

It has been suggested to me that these visual effects are indicative of photophobia, which is a migraine variant symptom. "Fear" and "overwhelming sense of vastness" may well relate to a spike of beta waves, 18 and 18.5 Hz. In the levels of 15 to 40 Hz intense anxiety and panic are induced.

REMOTE VIEWING

Due to the frequencies associated with the qualities of some crop circle's geometry and sound effects, even remote viewing can bring on extreme results. I had an email from a young woman who had an unexpected reaction to a picture of a crop circle.

> I looked at all the photos and studied the diagram that was presented on the site* in animated form. A few minutes later, I was sitting at my computer when I suddenly felt a bit dizzy. I got up from the chair and felt so woozy that I needed to lie down.
>
> My seven-year-old was quite concerned. I wanted a nap, but couldn't bear to shut out my child. Suddenly my stomach felt queasy as well. I was really frightened because I was so afraid something was seriously wrong with me, as I have never felt dizziness like that in my life, except for on an amusement ride!
>
> After a few runs to the bathroom, it suddenly occurred to me that perhaps it was brought on by the crop circle diagram/image. It's been six hours since it happened, and I still feel a tad dizzy, but not as much.

I suggested she should try and look at the images again without feeling that something would happen to her. She replied saying:

> I would certainly try to do what you suggest and look at the images again, but I'm actually afraid to do so! It was such an awful feeling! To be honest with you, I almost feel as though I can't bear to look at any images of crop formations without feeling extremely uneasy.

---

*cropcircles.lucypringle.co.uk/photos/2008/uk2008aa.shtml.

It's like when you have had a nightmare and can't bear to see the images resurface in your mind. Where before I could stare at the circles all day and get nothing but good feeling from them. Perhaps that particular formation, which possibly brought on the ill feelings (the April 19, 2008, Waden Hill formation), was a negatively formed/charged one?

It almost brings on a panicky feeling when I even just go to the website with the prospect of checking it out again. I can't bear to do it! Bizarre, I tell you. If and when I do study it again, I'll be sure to let you know what transpired, if I don't fall flat on the floor!

Later I received this encouraging email.

I have good news . . . I finally got the nerve to check out the pictures and diagram of the April 19 circle for the second time, taking your advice to do so, while thinking to myself that it won't affect me in any way.

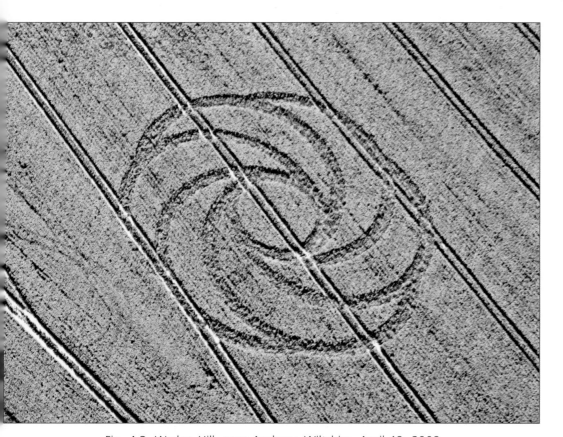

Fig. 4.3. Waden Hill, near Avebury, Wiltshire, April 19, 2008

This was about ten minutes ago, and whereas the last dizzying effects came upon me almost immediately after studying the photos and diagram when I looked at it for the first time on May 4, so far nothing feels out of the ordinary. And this time I spent more time on the site, and really concentrated on the photos and diagram.

NEW MEANING

The pleasure some people find in looking at crop circle photographs is very evident from the following email.

I've been meaning to contact you about an experience I had while meditating on the crop circle pictures in your book *Crop Circles: Art in the Landscape*. I find that gazing at pictures of crop circles brings on a very meditative state for me, and I love to use your book because there isn't a lot of text to distract me, and the photos are stunning.

I was looking at the pictures on page 37 . . . and I was thinking . . . I wonder what these really are . . . what are they for? And a voice—it was in my head, but not of my own thoughts—said, "They are didactic crosses."

I was taken aback and quickly took a notebook and wrote down the word *didactic* . . . because I had never heard it before and didn't know what it meant. So off to the computer to Google it. And I got chills when I read the meaning: "*didactic*: designed or intended to teach. Intended to convey instruction and information as well as pleasure and entertainment."

Now isn't that beautiful? Instruction, information, teaching, and pleasure looking at them, entertainment going into them and studying them. How perfect is that for a compact word to describe the circles?

NO WHEELCHAIR

The following is an extract of a report dictated to me by Paddy Lyons who, owing to her osteoarthritis, finds it too painful to write.

In October 2016 I received an invitation (as I do annually) from Lucy Pringle to attend her annual lecture in Petersfield, Hampshire, on the crop circles of that season. I mentioned it to my daughter and how sad I was that I couldn't go, to which she replied, "I don't see why you shouldn't;

I am going to take you." (We have very little money so my husband and daughter clubbed together in order to stay at a hotel near Petersfield overnight.)

My daughter drove me down to Petersfield. Unfortunately I was going through a particularly painful period and, even when in my wheelchair, was in acute pain. We arrived at the hotel and I rested for an hour before going to the lecture. The lecture was such a treat, and without realizing it, I was gradually going into a similar state to the one I had first felt when I went into the circle in 1996 at Stonehenge, the one called the Julia Set. I had no recollection afterward of what Lucy actually said.

When the lecture was over, without thinking, I got up from my wheelchair (which had been left in the passageway outside the lecture hall) and, forgetting that it wasn't just an ordinary chair and that I needed it, walked across the lecture hall to speak to Lucy. When I reached her, I realized what had happened. I was in no pain but my muscles started to feel weak. However, I was so delighted and was able to stand and chat to Lucy for quite a few minutes (normally I can't stand long enough to even brush my teeth).

I turned to walk back to my wheelchair, as I was beginning to feel rather weak, but still no pain. I felt as though a miracle had happened. Unfortunately the beautiful experience didn't last very long, and by the middle of the night I was in acute pain again, which lasted several weeks.

Despite the physical pain, my mood continued to feel radiant and at peace with the world and more able to tolerate my disability.

Many times I went into crop circles during the 1990s, and in early 2000 I went in on crutches and came out carrying my crutches above my head.

I have known Paddy Lyons since the 1990s and have witnessed the progression and deterioration of her condition and her determination and courage in trying her very best to continue visiting the crop circles against all odds and in severe pain. She loved flying over the circles as well as visiting them.

The above report is testimony of her courage. It was a humbling experience taking down her words as she dictated them in a factual, accepting, and uncomplaining manner in the face of great adversity and pain.

Relating to the October 2016 Petersfield lecture event, I was *astounded* to find Paddy standing waiting to talk to me after my lecture, no wheelchair, and standing as straight as a die. Her daughter, on the other hand, was darting around in a panic, thinking her mother was going collapse or fall at any moment. We talked for some time and Paddy confirmed that over 90 percent of the pain had gone. After a few minutes, she walked back across the large lecture hall, still straight-backed and walking like any normal person, and out of the hall. I stood quite still for some time afterward, trying to take in what I had just witnessed.

Paddy told me that she is due to have a shoulder replacement that will make getting around on her crutches even more difficult. Also as one of her ankles is beyond having a replacement, she is going to be having an L-shaped metal rod inserted in her foot and leg, immobilizing her ankle permanently but relieving the pain. Some people might question the sense of having all these seemingly endless and ghastly operations, but if you suffer the degree of pain that Paddy Lyons endures, to be rid of the acute pain is paramount on her agenda.

It is interesting to note that she had no remembrance of what I had talked about in my lecture, especially my report of how certain circles affected people to the extent that the frequencies emanating from them could be healing. One particular circle is not necessarily universally beneficial as we each respond to crop circles on a personal level. A circle that may be beneficial to one person may not have the same effect on others.

Another interesting point is that Paddy's symptoms seemed to worsen after the apparent temporary healing. This unfortunately has been reported on several occasions. To date we have no satisfactory medical explanation for these reports. The research continues.

A WONDERFUL GIFT

My final story is a happy one that may or may not be a result of a crop circle visit. Jennifer Denning, a watercolor artist, who kindly sent me this report, is firmly of the opinion that her cure is a result of her visit to the Mayan Calendar formation that appeared on the crest of the slope opposite Silbury Hill in August 2004.

The week before I had been given a picture taken from a newspaper of an enormous crop formation . . . which could not be seen from the road, but only after you had climbed up for about a quarter of a mile, to the crest of a large field. And there it was!! What a marvelous awe-inspiring image, which for my son and myself has proved to be both a revelation and

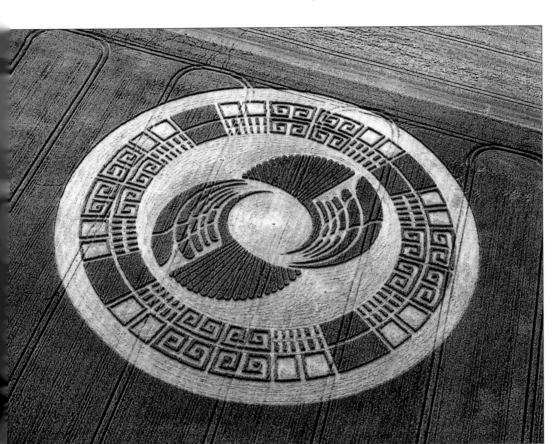

Fig. 4.4. Mayan Calendar, Silbury Hill, near Beckhampton, Wiltshire, August 3, 2004.

vibration-raising experience—and I believe was the start of the experiences to come later.

There was a downside to our visit to this formation. We both experienced headaches on the way home and felt extremely tired. I fell asleep easily, but was awoken at 1:00 a.m. with terrible pains down the left side of my body. It felt as if my body was contorted with cramps, and the pain in my left thigh drew my leg backward and upward quite violently and then spread downward to my left foot and upward into the groin and hip area. The pain was intense and continuous, and nothing I did helped to alleviate it. I could not move from the bed, and then a rigor set in, my teeth were chattering, and I shook uncontrollably for about ten minutes. Just as my husband was about to dial 999, it stopped—as suddenly as a light switch being turned off. The next day I felt totally drained, exhausted, and nauseous, but not bruised in any way as one usually does from cramps.

I called my son, Jonathan, about 11:00 a.m., and he told me that he had experienced a bad night also, with lots of joint pain, but fortunately not so severe, and that both the children were fine.

One of the most amazing things after this experience was the wonderful feeling of well-being and contentment that gradually spread through my being, and the ensuing happiness, which is still with me.

The most amazing thing is that I have also experienced a spontaneous healing of the eye problem that I had been suffering from. Macular degeneration had been diagnosed after I started having vision problems in late 2003.* Vision from my right eye was difficult, as I had distorted vision with all straight lines appearing wavy. This made reading difficult, and I was told on my last visit to the specialist in the autumn that it was progressive and I would probably need an operation. I was offered an operation at the Heath Hospital in Cardiff, which could take place before Christmas. After considering the verdict something made me ask if I could delay this and make another decision in January 2005 when I had my next appointment. This was agreed to reluctantly by the eye specialist, with instructions that if my sight worsened I was to come back to the hospital immediately.

However, one morning in early October I looked out the bedroom window thinking what a lovely day it was, and then suddenly realized that my eyesight was normal! No wavy lines! What a wonderful gift.

February 2005: Since writing this I have seen my eye specialist at the Royal Glamorgan Hospital, and he could see for himself the improvement in my vision. He said that he was surprised and that medically I was "a great rarity." Proof, if more were needed, that something happened that day in Wiltshire.

Further note, June 2005: I had an eye test with my usual optician and she told me that my reading vision had also improved.

In July 2005 I again attended the Crop Circle Symposium, which is when I spoke to you, Lucy, and showed you the photos of the beautiful orbs that have been appearing in my photos, and also spoke about the healing of my eye problem.

You asked me to contact you after seeing the eye specialist in September, hence this letter. I have my appointment letter if you wish to see it.

---

*Research by the Mayo Foundation explains macular degeneration at www.mayoclinic.org.

September 2005: I have seen an eye specialist again at the RGH, and once again he could not account for the improvement in my sight. The next appointment will now be in eight months' time, which, he said, is just to monitor the situation. My sight is still fine, and every day I am aware of the wonderful gift that I have been given.

I hope my experience will prove useful to you in your research, I do strongly believe that the energy held in these formations can be transformational.

COMMENTS BY JAMES LYONS

Crop circles, just like every scenario in the Cosmos, are defined in terms of waves. Just as we see ripples on a pond or ocean waves, these waves can be either stationary or moving as on water.

Waves are defined by two parameters. The first is the wavelength, that is, the length of one complete cycle, which is defined by one up and one down motion. The second parameter is the frequency of the wave. This is the number of cycles we observe usually in one second. Thus we are all used to tuning in to TV and radio programs. Each such program covers a band of frequencies, the whole spectrum being termed a channel.

In everyday life, we mostly experience light waves, which our eyes clearly tune in to. The rainbow demonstrates the different combination of colors to which different cone structures in our eyes are tuned.

However, when we refer to other waves such as sound, then the frequencies involved are far lower than light. Indeed the band of frequencies varies from a few cycles per second, which we perceive as rumbles, up to around 20 kHz (thousands of cycles per second). The ability to hear this top frequency regrettably reduces with age.

Now, sound waves possess a totally different structure from light waves. Whereas the latter are essentially electric in nature, they combine with an associated magnetic wave to create, not surprisingly, electromagnetic waves. They are indeed the structure of light, which possesses a maximum speed. Sound waves are all to do with longitudinal waves, that is, waves that oscillate back and forth.

The clearest way to grasp the difference between these two forms of wave motion is to envisage a Slinky toy. The electromagnetic wave is akin to shaking the Slinky up and down, whereas pulling it like a concertina generates sound waves. Whereas the former is purely electrical in nature and operates in a

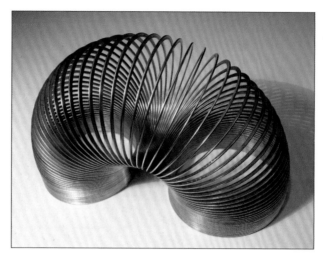

Fig. 4.5. The Slinky.

vacuum, sound waves require the medium of air to travel through. No air, no sound waves.

There is one rather unique type of wave that is not even well known in mainstream science. This is the so-called torsion wave. If we consider a Slinky toy again, then the motion is a twisting one. This oscillating rotational movement is key to virtually all long-distance cosmic connectivity.

Light takes a little over eight minutes to reach Earth from the Sun. This is pathetically slow for communication even to our outer Solar System. Torsion waves travel at a speed that is 10^{39} times faster. These types of electric waves are key to intergalactic communication. They are termed Birkeland currents and were first found over a hundred years ago. Everyone is familiar with them, usually unbeknown to us, since in acoustic form, they are the sounds generated by all bowed instruments such as violins, cellos, and so forth. The bow twists the string, which vibrates in a twisting motion.

Why do frequencies occur in crop circles? Every pattern is in fact made up of signals of differing frequencies. We are all used to looking at newspapers, TVs, and computer screens. These images are in fact nothing but a matrix of dots, which these days are mostly colored as per rainbows. However, in Earth Energy patterns, it is usual to find the waves, which create the images, are primarily represented during crop circle creation as waves surrounding energy structures. The primary shape is that of a ring. The creation process is like a smoker blowing smoke rings. These rings, to use the technical term, are *toroids*. The toroid and the sphere are the fundamental topological structures of space.

The Platonic solids are fundamental geometrical forms derived from the two topological structures—e.g., a cube nested within a sphere. They are subsets of the two topological structures.

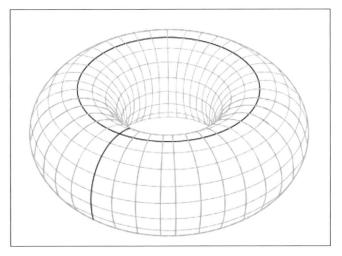

Fig. 4.6. The torus.

Now imagine our Slinky toy being joined at its ends, thus creating a ring but clearly having wave structures around it. This form occurs everywhere in the Cosmos. As described in more detail in the appendices, this energy form "emerges" from the earth where a crop circle is formed. These bubble rings rise to the surface and are created from electric strikes to underground water sources. Like bubbles in water, they rise to the surface, and on breaking through, just as soap bubbles pop, so do these wave rings of energy. The collapsing bubble with its significantly lower pressure inside than outside "sucks down" the crop in a very controlled manner. The result for such a simple form is clearly a circle.

Thus, in essence, a crop circle is a "frozen-in-time" wave. The size of the circle depends on the depth from which it is generated and the angle of the cone, which dictates how the cone size grows in moving to the surface. It turns out that the frequencies involved in the creation process are very low, of the order at most of a few cycles per second, not unlike earthquakes. The wave velocity again is low, of the order of a few feet per second. This process has been observed by those lucky enough to see one forming.

By contrast, the electrical phenomena involved are often directly visible in the form of both spiraling columns of energy, akin to a vertical Slinky-toy wave motion. In addition, small balls of light are sometimes seen moving along the energy lines associated with the basic grid layout of the formation. Plasma phenomena are not always visible, since in addition to the glow mode associated with plasmas, there are also arc modes and indeed dark modes, the most common form in Earth Energy activities. The triggering force is electrical in nature, but its strikes to Earth release what are essentially acoustic waves from underground water. Pattern formation is a repeated version of this fundamental process.

As indicated, we have to differentiate between the frequencies involved by measurement either of the pattern-wave structure, readily undertaken with tape measures, or by using meters of various kinds. Crop circles can create ambient waves, which are retained within the creation electrical double layer, which forms the overall energy hemisphere. These can be detected though not always measured, using electrostatic detection meters. As there are many types on the market, it is not always straightforward to detect, measure, and classify such electrostatic fields. This task is often undertaken at stone circles where similar energy fields are far more stable and columnar vortices are detectable at nodal points on the Earth-grid system.

5

CROP CIRCLE GEOMETRY AND MUSIC

The mathematician's patterns, like the painter's or the poet's, must be beautiful; the ideas, like the colours or the words, must fit together in a harmonious way.

GODFREY HAROLD HARDY, FRS (1877–1947)

OCCASIONALLY, PERMANENT HEALING occurs as a result of visiting crop circles, but, as we discussed earlier, the majority of reports fall into the list of negative effects; crop circle visitors automatically expect to feel well and therefore are surprised and dismayed when the opposite occurs.

However, whereas the greater numbers of healing events are unfortunately only temporary in nature, they are still worth discussing in order to illustrate the effects of the inherent residual "energies" at the sites and their subsequent impact on living systems, even from a distance.

Pythagoras was the first to recognize that music and numbers were linked, and as we look at images of crop circles we will notice that many are shaped like mandalas. As all genuine crop circles are based on geometry, the geometric figures are emitting frequencies just as Pythagoras described, thus stimulating our brains and resulting in various different mental or physical reactions.

Mandalas are the schematic representations of the Cosmos in Buddhist, Native American, and other traditions. Seen as universal symbols, they were used by our ancient forebears to induce meditative and trancelike states. Just as a musical chord can activate resonances in the ear and the brain, which kindle emotions, mandalas can also affect people who view them. This effect is known as a "sign stimulus," and it triggers a behavioral response without requiring knowledge or understanding on the part of the person. All mandalas contain certain essential geometric principles, such as number, form, and ratio; many are based on Platonic solids and are rooted in sacred geometry.

Sacred geometry teaches us that buildings containing these geometric principles and proportions are more harmonious and remedial. Our ancient cathedrals all observe and are true to this fundamental geometry, and if this idea were carried forward to our schools and hospitals, I feel certain the benefits would be recognized and more widely implemented.

On one occasion I was giving a talk in New York and the hall was filling up but not everyone was seated; a girl arrived and rebuked me for starting late. I smiled at her and said that I hoped she would receive what she needed from my talk. Afterward she came up to me transformed. She apologized for being rude and explained that she had had a long-term painful knee and that during my talk the pain had completely disappeared. Unfortunately I did not get her contact details so was unable to follow up her case.

Many people are extremely sensitive to these transmitted energies; some people find that they are unable to look at pictures of certain formations, while others feel nausea or appear to fall asleep.

On another occasion I was giving an early morning talk at the Harry Edwards Healing Centre in Surrey. During the talk not only was a strange ticking sound heard by many (there was no clock in the room, the central heating was not on, nor were there any workmen around), but a couple of people, much to their chagrin, fell asleep during the talk. "I have never fallen asleep so early in the morning," said one.

After the talk we sat outside and chatted about many things including the ticking, and I heard one of the slumberers say, "O yes, I remember that." I had observed her sleeping at that particular time! It seems that whereas the person appears to all intents and purposes to be asleep, they are only in an induced "mandala" trancelike state and can indeed hear everything!

THE HARP

May 2009 was a glorious month. The Sun shone and circles appeared—one clearly depicting a musical instrument. Therefore I was delighted to receive an email from Dr. Karen Ralls, a medieval historian at the University of

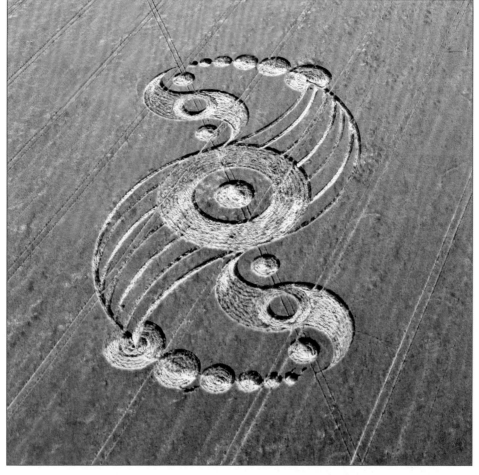

Fig. 5.1. The Harp at Windmill Hill, Wiltshire, May 25, 2009. An elaborate
formation consisting of a center circle with two large and two
small arcs extended and connected by circles of decreasing size.
Once again seems to follow the yin yang theme.

Edinburgh, and a longtime music researcher into the history of ancient and wooden flutes.

A postgraduate student had mentioned my website to Dr. Ralls, suggesting that she might like to have a look at the Windmill Hill Harp imagery, and the symbolism regarding the number seven, in general.

In her email Dr. Ralls explained,

Regarding the number seven, the overall situation is rather complex, but fascinating. It is a theme many have explored over the years in a variety of ways.

It seems that at the very beginning (i.e., in the West), among the objects created by pre-Greek inhabitants of the Aegean area in general, the earliest known stringed instrument is the harp.

In fact, last night I was learning more about the early visual depictions of at least seven small marble figures of seated harpists that belong to the period between about 2700 and 2100 BCE. These were discovered on islands in the Cyclades—Keros, Thera, and Naxos.

The instruments tend to be referred to by earlier musicologists as the "Cycladic harps"—but the precise language or culture of these people is still little known. However, in time, more information will probably come to light from archaeologists.

Some of the archaeologists believe that (as the figures were pre-Greek), they may possibly have come from west Anatolia (modern Turkey) and then into the Aegean/Greek areas.

Since these marble figures don't show the exact number of strings or how they were plucked, etc., it cannot be known how many strings there were for sure. There is a general lack of sources from about 2000 to 1500 BCE, and it is not at present certain exactly what cultural contacts there were between these early Cycladic people and the Greek-speaking people who began to arrive in the Aegean area after 2000 BCE.

Of course, as more research from many fields comes to light in the future, the overall picture will become much clearer.

In addition, I found that on counting the smaller circles on the outside of the harp there were 19. The number 19 has been found in stone circles in the British Isles and is thought to relate to the nineteen-year Metonic cycle.

Meton was a Greek mathematician and astronomer who lived in Athens in the fifth century BCE. Meton found that nineteen solar years are almost equal to 235 lunar months and 6940 days. The nineteen-year Metonic lunisolar calendar was named after him.

THE DECIMAL, THE FRACTION, AND THE OGHAM ALPHABET

In 2008 a truly remarkable event occurred on June 1. A curious signature appeared in one of the fields lying beneath the famous Barbury Castle Iron Age Hill Fort in Wroughton on the northern edge of the Wiltshire Downs.

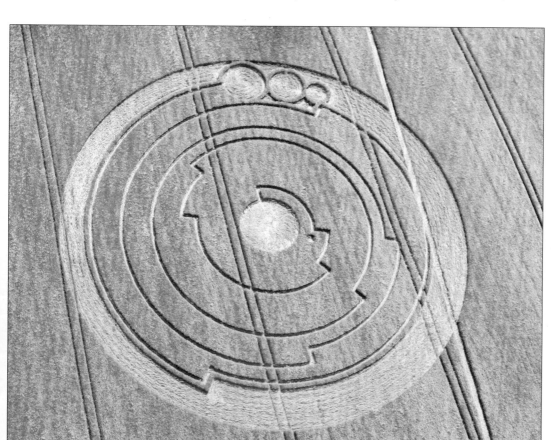

Fig. 5.2. Barbury Castle, Wroughton, Wiltshire, June 1, 2008.

It is thought that the Barbury Castle site was first occupied going back some 2,500 years, and at that time was in use during the Roman occupation of the area. Archaeological investigations at Barbury have shown evidence of a number of buildings indicating a village or military garrison located there. Once the battleground of the Saxons against the Britons in 556 CE, it rightfully boasts fantastic views over the surrounding countryside.

The crop circle was undoubtedly the pick of the season, covering some twelve acres. Flying over it shortly after it appeared it seemed an unusual series of ratchets and circles within a circular frame. Posting my images on the internet, I received an email from retired astrophysicist Mike Reed who had seen my images on Linda Moulton Howe's excellent website (www.earthfiles.com).

Reed has impeccable references, having worked at the University of Arizona in Tucson on the Multiple Mirror Telescope (MMT) at Mount

Hopkins, a joint venture with the Harvard Smithsonian Observatory. He told me,

> I noticed the Barbury Castle pattern posted on the Earthfiles site yesterday. It is apparently a coded image representing the first ten digits of Pi (the ratio of the circumference of a circle to the diameter). The tenth digit has even been correctly rounded up. The little dot near the center is the decimal point.
>
> The attached diagram [Mike Reed kindly allowed me to make the diagram slightly clearer, and Andreas Mueller then finished it professionally] shows the analysis that reveals the code [see fig. 5.3]. It is based on ten angular segments with the radial jumps being the indicator of each segment. Starting at the center and counting the number of 1/10 segments in each section contained by the change in radius clearly shows the values of the first ten digits in the value of Pi.

James Lyons commented,

> Pi = 3.141592654, to ten places rounded up. The actual value to twelve places is 3.14159265358. You can see that the tenth digit has been rounded up from 3 to 4 since the next digit is a 5.
>
> The three circles at the top to the right of the top four just under the perimeter are not circles, or spheres or ellipses; they are an ellipsis, the geometric term for "and so on," which exactly characterized Pi!
>
> Is there any evidence that this circle is man made? If not this is certainly an interesting development.

Longtime crop circle researcher Charles Mallett visited the formation on the morning after it had appeared and reported that there was no mud on the fallen crop. As it had rained that night his is an interesting comment, for when the soil is wet just walking down a tramline leaves us with soil building up on the soles of our shoes until it feels as though we are walking on stilts. It would have been humanly impossible to construct a formation in those conditions without leaving any trace of mud; indeed, I have been into several formations over the years in which the flattened crop has been covered in mud, which would suggest they were human made.

Not content with giving us a circle with Pi in decimal form, the phenomenon produced another earlier circle in fraction form. It was geometer Michael

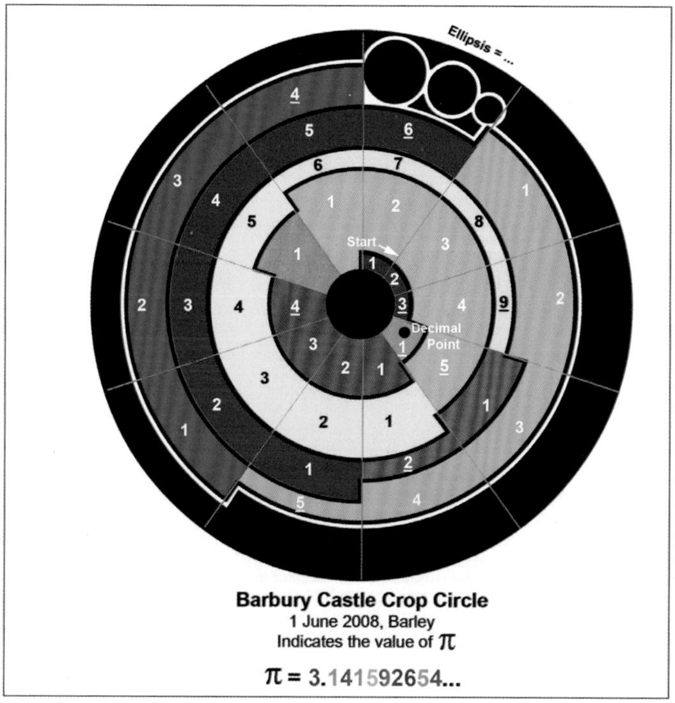

Fig. 5.3. A diagram of the Barbury Castle crop circle.

Glickman who made this discovery: "Several formations had referred to 22/7. Perhaps the most significant of these was Picked Hill (sometimes referred to as Woodborough Hill) of August 13, 2000, which again used both 44 radial and 14 concentric geometries [which divided by 2, gives us 22/7]. The brilliance of this exemplary crop circle is confirmed by the implicit heptagram, which restates the seven." Geometer Michael Glickman writes that

traditionally the square has represented the world and material realty while the circle has been the symbol of Heaven and Spirituality.

In the 90s the circles started referring to squaring the circle. This symbolises the marriage of Earth and Heaven, a bridge between Man and Spirit, and the circles, through their reiteration, seemed anxious to emphasize it.

Pi is the arithmetical constant used in all calculations involving circles and circularity. Pi might be read as a key to the door between circles and squares.

Pi, in its purest state, is an irrational or infinite number whose digits extend into many millions. It starts 3.141592 . . . and then continues forever. . . . Obviously this level of precision is rarely needed and so 22/7

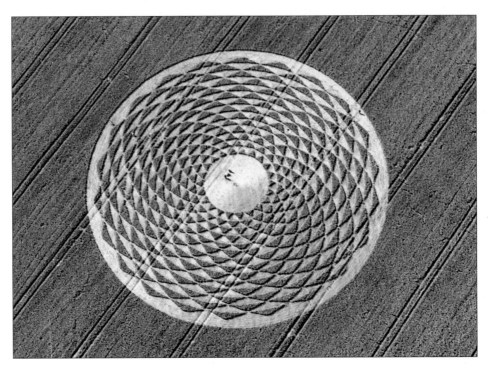

Fig. 5.4. Woodborough Hill, Woodborough, Wiltshire, August 13, 2000.

(3.142857 . . .) has been adopted as a close enough and more practical substitute.

The beautiful Woodborough Hill formation of August 13, 2000, was an outstanding example of 22/7. A circle can be divided in two ways: radially (that is divided from the center like a pizza) and concentrically (like ripples on the surface of water after a stone has been thrown in). Woodborough, radially, had 44 divisions. Were it a pizza, each of the forty four guests would have a ludicrously thin wedge of 8.1818 . . .° while concentrically it displayed 14 rings. Forty-four over fourteen is equal to 22/7 = Pi.

As explained previously, we were taught at school that Pi or π is a mathematical constant that represents the ratio of any circle's circumference to its diameter in Euclidean geometry, which is the same as the ratio of a circle's area to the square of its radius. Pi is one of the most important mathematical constants: many formulae from mathematics, science, and engineering involve Pi.

Surely there can be no clearer indication that we are dealing with an intelligence behind this phenomenon by producing formations showing us Pi in both decimal and fraction form?

Possibly one of the most teasing events of 2010 was the much-debated early formation at Wilton, Wiltshire, appearing beneath the famous windmill on May 22.

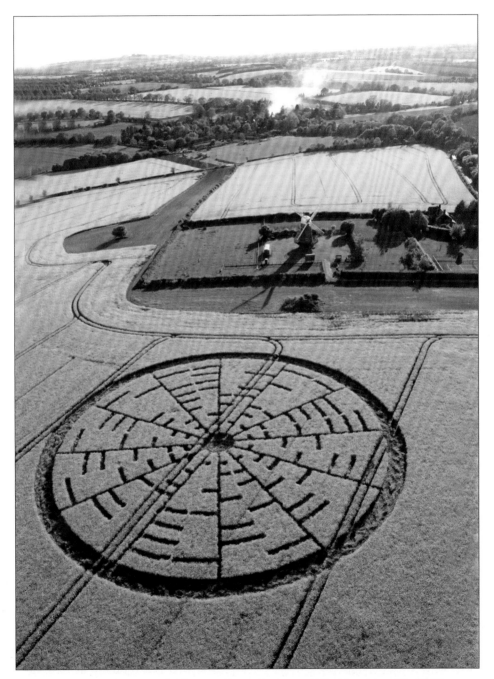

Fig. 5.5. Wilton Windmill, near Great Bedwyn, Wiltshire, May 22, 2010.

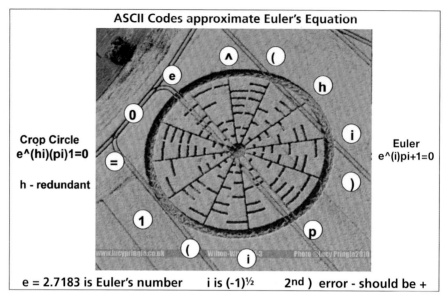

Fig. 5.6. The Wilton Windmill formation showing the Euler equation anomalies.

As with the earlier circles, it was in oilseed rape (canola). Some likened it to the ancient Ogham alphabet thought to have been brought here by the Celts who originally migrated from Assyria to Mesopotamia (Iraq) before arriving in Great Britain. Others preferred Russian-born physicist Leonhard Euler's equation, but, after close examination, it was clear that several anomalies existed as illustrated by James Lyons's excellent diagram, shown in figure 5.6, and his commentary just below. (Please refer to appendix 7, page 228, for more on the Wilton Windmill.)

> The small lines in the Wilton Windmill event resemble the Ogham alphabet which is thought to be named after the Irish god Ogma. The origins of the alphabet are unknown but the generally accepted opinion is that it could have been used as a system of tallies for accounting. Clearly only the inscriptions on stone remain as evidence, but it is likely that they were generally inscribed on sticks, stakes, or trees. We are told that the inscriptions would generally have taken the form of somebody's name and the name of a place and were probably used to mark boundaries.

These anomalies drew Linda Moulton Howe's attention to the German physicist Max Planck's theory of the Wave Structure of Matter (WSM) and Standing-Wave Interactions (which occur at discrete frequencies f), which

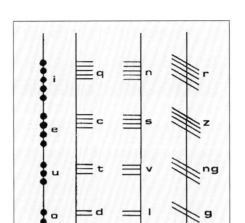

Fig. 5.7. The ancient Ogham alphabet.

explains Quantum Energy States of Matter and Light, "Quanta" ($E = hf$).*

Another interesting discovery by James Lyons was the presence of the diatonic ratio encoded in the design (white notes on the piano). Able to play it on his piano he told me, "it was not very harmonious." It was the late musicians Paul Vigay and David Kingston who were the first to transform the crop circle geometry into music with some quite remarkable results.

Having woken at 4:00 a.m. one morning and unable to get back to sleep, I decided to drive down to Wiltshire and see the formation for myself. It had been raining heavily overnight and despite having stopped by the time I arrived, I had forgotten how much water the yellow petals retain. The crop stood about five feet tall, and in no time at all I was drenched from head to toe, and my Wellingtons were full of water that had trickled relentlessly downward off my clothes. In addition, I had forgotten to bring my aerial photograph, and since the formation could not be seen from the ground (only from the air or the windmill and this had been closed the weekend the formation appeared), I simply could not find it and was getting wetter and wetter. Not surprisingly, not many people were happy to answer my early-morning mobile telephone calls until Julian Gibson nobly answered his and gave me the necessary directions. The

---

*For more on Planck's theory, see www.spaceandmotion.com/quantum-theory-max-planck-quotes.htm.

outer ring was much trampled and did not provide me with the information I needed. However, the lay of the crop was remarkable, lying in a crisscrossing herringbone manner. I made my way inward to areas that had been untouched and found what I was looking for, an unbroken stem without any cracks above or below. Canola snaps if bent an angle of 40 degrees; it also cracks and bruises very easily if any weight is applied, which would indicate it was man made or that people had previously visited the formation if several days old. That is why it is important to try to enter a circle almost as soon as it appears before

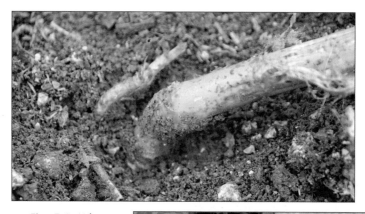

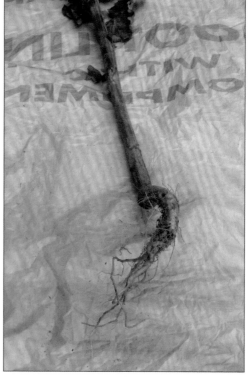

Fig. 5.8. **Above,** undamaged canola plant stem. **Right,** root to undamaged canola plant stem. Wilton Windmill, Great Bedwyn, Wiltshire, May 22, 2010.

any physical evidence is destroyed by visitors. In order to ascertain this properly, it is necessary to dig away the soil from some way down around the stem. Holding my camera with soil-covered, wet, and slippery hands, I managed to get a photograph. Now soaked to the skin, and hoping that no one was around, I did a quick strip, discarding first my sweater, replacing it with a jacket that came down to my knees and hid the fact that I had also discarded my jeans. Luckily I did not have to stop for anything on my way home so modesty was preserved! Definitely worth the effort.

COMMENTS BY JAMES LYONS

All animals, as we ourselves do, respond to vibrations of the air around them. In structured form we recognize the effect as music.

It is well known that the style of the music is critical to where it is heard or played and its intended purpose. Thus, it is not surprising, say, to hear a Schubert quartet in an old people's home, rather than a rock band. So what is it about music that literally resonates with us?

We know that, at best, we can only hear frequencies up to 20 kHz. This is way below bats, for example, who can hear to frequencies at least twice this value.

Air motion, such as a breeze, is of course a daily experience, but there are several scenarios in which air moves in a coordinated fashion. Putting aside wind in general, we must note severe events such as hurricanes and more local phenomena such as dust devils, which are vortex columns of air.

In crop circles, there are many events involving rotating columns of not only air but also embedded electrical phenomena. The frequencies of rotation are related to Earth-vibration effects. Of more immediate appearance are the patterns of the formations themselves.

It turns out that the underlying pattern of crop circles follows the grid of energy lines upon which, for example, medieval churches as well as ancient sites such as Stonehenge and Avebury were located. These so-called acupuncture points on the Earth are colloquially termed "spiders' webs" since in the UK they usually comprise six rings with eight radial lines. They are located at the crossover of telluric currents within the ground, the centerlines being located at the center of the formation.

It is the vibration of the Earth currents that creates the patterns. This process is well known, and imitation formations can be created in a dish holding a layer of sand. Sound generators not unlike loudspeakers below the dish, on being activated by specific frequencies cause the sand to move laterally to congregate at the nodal points within the dish. By combining different frequencies, the collective harmonic pattern can produce an incredible variety of shapes. We have noted that the basic creation mechanism of crop circles is from below via rising toroidal shapes. It is the modulation frequencies on these toroids that define basic patterns. A more detailed discussion of the diatonic scale can be found in appendix 7.

Thus, summarizing the music-to-brain-wave connection we find in crop circles, we can say with some confidence that brain frequencies align with natural frequencies in formation. What the ambient vibrational energy in the circles is doing is totally analogous to an oboist tuning up an orchestra. Thus out-of-tune brain waves are entrained to function at their intended frequencies. In other words, this is Mother Nature's way of retuning the brain to its natural state.

In specific formations, the multi-circle spiral formation, the Julia Set (1996), which took around thirty minutes to form, is perhaps the most forceful example of the harmonic sequence in operation. An eyewitness account of this event is found in appendix 1, pages 204–5.

From a simple center circle, we see that the creating energy, initially rising as a simple toroidal form in the center, then rises to the shell energy dome and returns back to Earth, this time not creating a circle but, seeing it is essentially a long tapering cone of spiraling energy, it reemerges, smaller in size in a differing predetermined location. This process is repeated, thus creating the tapering arms, which slowly rotate each new circle to form the arms. Each individual circle in itself has a rotating ring from which smaller side circles are formed.

Of all the formations that have been created since the early 1990s, this one must qualify as the key teacher for demonstrating the underlying creation process. This reveals in particular three key facets of the crop circle phenomenon.

1. It highlights basics of simple circle creation from below.
2. It most clearly demonstrates the harmonic sequence involved.
3. Having been seen forming, it revealed to many not only the crop circle creation process but also the cosmic processes of Galaxy creation.

From the health perspective, the separately tuned circles resonate with the neural structure of the brain and show how in principle crop circle energy yields the synergistic energy fields, which can realign or retune the human being's fundamental harmonic structure.

6

TECHNICAL AND MECHANICAL FAILURES

Science is organized knowledge. Wisdom is organized life.

IMMANUEL KANT (1724–1804)

THE EVER-INCREASING USE OF, and exposure to, electrical equipment and electrical fields that are stronger than those that occur in the natural environment are inevitably causing a disturbing disruption to our well-being, and more serious in-depth research is needed in this highly sensitive and controversial area. The equipment that produce these fields include such items as microwave ovens, mobile telephones, computers, the internet, washing machines, refrigerators, air conditioners, electric blankets, televisions, hairdryers, and so forth. The results of these effects are playing an integral part in our daily existence; we are in fact bombarded with these higher frequencies every day of our lives, and the consequences of these fields on our central nervous system must be an area of concern.

Paul Vigay was one of the first people to experience and record electrical anomalies. He found that, on numerous occasions, his mobile phone would not work when inside the circle but would operate perfectly when outside the circle. He would repeat this several times with exactly the same effect.

He developed his first detection gizmo in 1990. He had been experimenting with some electrical components, and the net result was Mark One, which was initially designed to pick up weak electrical currents such as those coming from light switches and cables. I remember him demonstrating it along the walls in my house and it seemed to work pretty well. I was most impressed!

One day he was at his parents' house. His mother, Mavis, had visited a crop circle and had hung several bunches of wheat taken from the crop circle in the kitchen to dry. Paul had been idly playing around with his gadget when he decided to test it against these bundles of wheat and was amazed at the different signals he got. One bunch gave a very strong reading whereas the other didn't.

On asking Mavis about them he realized that it was the samples taken from inside the crop circle that were giving the strong reading, while the others gave no reaction whatsoever. Whatever the "energy" is, it clearly can remain active for some time after the event.

HE HAD TO CHANGE HIS MIND

Strange and unexpected events occur not only to humans and animals while inside or in the vicinity of crop circles but also to inanimate objects such as farm machinery and electrical devices.

I was doing a television interview in 1997 on a newly discovered circle at Milk Hill in Wiltshire. The farmer and owner of the field, Brian Reid, joined us and all was going happily and smoothly until the program producer asked the farmer to harvest out the formation by driving his harvester through the center of the circle so that they could capture this event on camera.

I was horrified and protested loudly and vehemently—"it is like cutting the center piece out of the Mona Lisa; you can't do that," I cried. All to no avail: the farmer got into his harvester and *clankety-clank, clankety-clank* went the monstrous machine.

I could not bear to watch; this was sacrilege, I turned my back on the scene and closed my eyes. Closer and closer came the sound until—suddenly silence. I turned round, and to my utter delight, the harvester had broken down.

The toolbox was produced, spanners appeared, and sadly within minutes the fault was mended and again with my back turned I could hear the dreaded *clankety-clank, clankety-clank* as it drew closer and closer until yet again—sudden silence. Joy of joys, the harvester had broken down for the second time just before reaching the circle. What was happening? The farmer looked bewildered.

Out came the toolbox and more spanners and other gear flew around until the harvester reluctantly started, and before I knew it the center of the formation was stripped bare. I was horrified by such desecration.

It was only the following year when I bumped into Brian Reid that he came up to me and took me to one side. He confided that never before had his

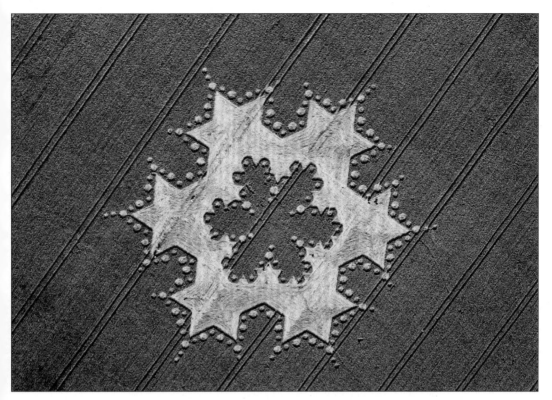

Fig. 6.1. Milk Hill, Alton Barnes, Wiltshire, August 7, 1997.

machinery failed, and not just once but twice. He said that previously he had always believed that all the circles were man made but had had to change his mind after this experience!

The next sections are devoted to electrical anomalies where the number of reports are so enormous that once more there is a need to be selective.

THEY CAME BACK TO LIFE

It was a little too dark to take photos without a flash, but I thought I would try anyway (I knew the battery in my camera was flat; it had been for some time). I started to take photos and the flash worked. I looked at the battery indicator at the top of my camera and it registered a full battery.

Later that morning I met a friend, and we went to my local photographic shop where my batteries were certified dead. I bought replacements but retained my old ones. Returning home exhausted later that evening, I resolved that if I did nothing else before tumbling into bed, I must test my "dead" batteries. I put them back in my cameras and, lo and behold, they were as strong as if they were new. I have used them ever since!

When we entered the Telegraph Hill formation that morning, a friend had laid his second camera (Nikon FM 5 volt, using FUJI Super G ASA 200) on the ground while he assembled his pole and took several shots of the formation.

When he had finished he collected the Nikon that had been lying on the ground and walked up the tramline at the top of the formation. The light meter glowed dimly a few times and faded completely. The battery was dead. Fortunately he had not thrown out his old batteries and I suggested he should retain and test them. He rang me the following day to tell me that his defunct batteries had also come back to life!

Another visitor to the circle said, "I thought I would take a picture from this formation looking up at the hill we had just sat on, but when I tried the camera, which has an electronic 'wind-on,' I found there was no life in it at all, which was strange because it had been functioning perfectly prior to this moment. It did not come back to life until I was back in the car."

2000

Dr. Richard Boylan informs us that, when flying over a formation that had appeared on August 14 in a field of wheat at the corner of 93 South and Church Drive, between Whitefish and Kalispell, Montana, the pilot noticed his compass sway 10 degrees. "I had just recharged my new eight-hour camcorder battery. But after taping for only twenty minutes, the battery was drained."

Research immunologist Dr. Roger Taylor sent this report:

We were in a crop circle on Hackpen Hill, the first of August, with some American friends. Their camera would not focus properly, so that they were unable to take any pictures. On taking it to the shop, it turned out the battery (which had been almost new) was flat. After getting a new battery, they were able to take pictures in other crop circles, but there was still a residual problem with the autofocus.

Roger has a very sensitive and advanced program using computerized Kirlian photography, which sends a high-voltage discharge from his finger to the electrode. He refused to take it into any crop formations for fear of costly electrical disturbance to the equipment.

In the three-segmented formation at Liddington Castle a brand new camcorder with two new batteries had complete battery failure within two minutes.

I had brought my Sony digital video camera and taped extensively, using special effects. At one point I laid my camera on the ground in the center of one of the small circles and immediately remembered Ron Russell telling me how he had done the same one time and had damaged his camera. I snatched it up, but too late; my eight-hour $150 battery was dead, and I could not recharge it fully. It read strangely on my equipment—"full" on the camera, but "three hours" on the charger, no matter how long I left it to charge. I have two batteries and the other one, which was left in the room, was normal.

1998

A colleague from the Wiltshire Group relates how in 1998, when she did a radio interview in the formation opposite Silbury Hill on Tuesday morning, May 5, for the local station, the tape sped up so considerably that it appeared

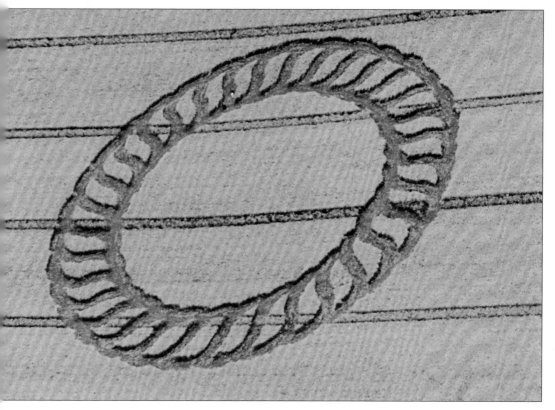

Fig. 6.2. Silbury Beltane Wheel, near Beckhampton, Wiltshire, May 4, 1998.

to stop. Being accustomed to electrical failures inside formations, she suggested they take the tape machine outside the formation. At a distance of about fifty yards from the formation the tape machine worked perfectly. They repeated this test several times with identical results. The interview was played over the radio without cutting the bizarre sound effects; it sounded like gobbledygook as the tape sped up. The interviewer, who had previously been a skeptic, was taken aback by these unexplained events, events that she has never experienced before; she is now convinced that this is a genuine phenomenon and wanted everyone to hear the strange recording!

This is not the end of the story. Later in the day, Western Television also visited the formation. They were even more skeptical, pooh-poohing the whole subject and indicating that anyone who believed the formations were other than man made were either stupid or gullible.

My colleague longed for something strange to occur and wished her very deepest wish that some anomaly would convince them otherwise, but as the time wore on and nothing untoward had happened, she was despondent but resigned. That evening the pictures were shown on the local television with brief reporter coverage.

The next morning a member of the television technical crew telephoned to say that the reason the reported coverage had been so short was because their sound system had been so disrupted that most of the recording was unusable. He simply could not understand this; their sound equipment was of the very highest quality and the most reliable available, designed to cope with any situation. It had never failed before!

A man who visited the 2002 formation called the Druids' Knot, Alton Priors, on the first morning took four camera batteries with him. Three were newly charged rechargeable batteries; the fourth was a completely new non-rechargeable battery. To his dismay he was only able to take four pictures as one by one the batteries drained as soon as he put them into his camera.

I visited this formation with meteorologist Alan Day the morning it appeared. He was keen to help me bury my bottles. I was walking ahead of him and suddenly heard him say "Oh no!" followed a few seconds later by "Oh damn!" Turning around I found him gazing in fury at his camera. He had only shot five or six frames when the camera went forward two frames and then within seconds whizzed the whole way back into the canister, taking the tab with it.

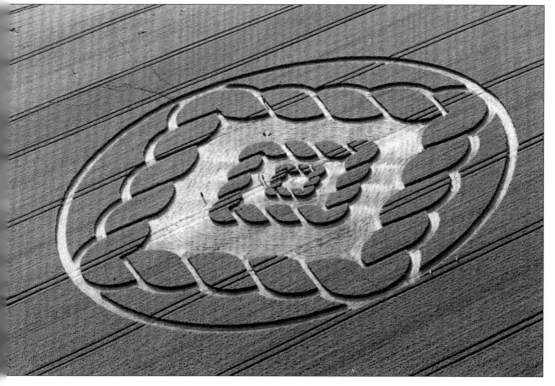

Fig. 6.3. The Druids' Knot, Alton Priors, Wiltshire, July 22, 2002.

A few days later I did an interview with an Italian TV company. I happened to mention this incident to the cameraman whose eyes lit up as I related the story; his camera had failed in the exact same spot. It had never happened to him before. Fortunately it recovered when he moved off to another area of the formation.

Camera and mobile-telephone failures are almost too numerous to mention. However, this anomaly can be extremely annoying especially when flying, and when the camera fails just as one has eventually managed to get the formation perfectly within the frame.

Crop circles have often been the plague of my life, as I have lost count of the number of times when I have had the perfect image in the frame and was just about to take the picture, when, lo and behold, the camera button would not depress—or even worse, one time the whole image seemed to be cut in two, only to find that when flying away from the circle, the camera functioned perfectly. We would return to the circle and the same glitch would occur. We repeated it several more times only to give up in the end. Grrrr!

Camera malfunctions have happened to me on many occasions, but this one particular time, when flying over the newly formed three-sided scalloped formation containing nested crescents at the Sanctuary, was especially irksome. The clouds had momentarily disappeared, and I had clear sunlit visibility and perfect positioning. All to no avail, my camera containing slide film would not focus. Try as I might by putting it on every conceivable setting, it still refused to focus. Yet another broken camera!

In my frustration, I felt like tossing it into the beyond. However, good sense prevailed and we set off to photograph another formation using my other camera with print film. On our return I happened to pick up the rogue camera and lo and behold it focused perfectly.

I KNEW MY BATTERY WAS FULLY CHARGED

Reports of mechanical and battery failures abound. Valerie Charlton visited the Wansdyke in Wiltshire on August 26, 2001, to see the Milk Hill formation when it was two weeks old. She reported:

I have a Canon UC9 Hi8 Camcorder, which I have used for the past four years, without it ever failing to work. I have two available batteries, one large (Duracell DR12, 6V), which will easily last for three hours of filming, and a smaller one that lasts about half an hour. I charged up the large battery overnight and put it on the camera before leaving Midhurst to drive to Wiltshire at about 11:00 a.m. I did not take the smaller one (Canon battery pack, BP-711, 6V, 1100mAh Ni-Cd battery) with me, knowing I was unlikely to film for more than three hours.

As I walked up the formation on the track I took out the camera meaning to film the wonderful view of the land dropping away to the right of Milk Hill, thinking it would describe the landscape in which the crop circle had occurred. The camera would not work no matter what I did. I tried taking the battery off the camera several times in case it hadn't engaged properly. The red light on the camera would not function.

I was very irritated and disappointed, but, because I knew the battery was fully charged I just thought that my camera must have been damaged, it didn't occur to me at the time that the crop circle might have drained my battery.

When I got home I put in the smaller battery and the camera worked perfectly. I then put the bigger battery on charge overnight and in the morning

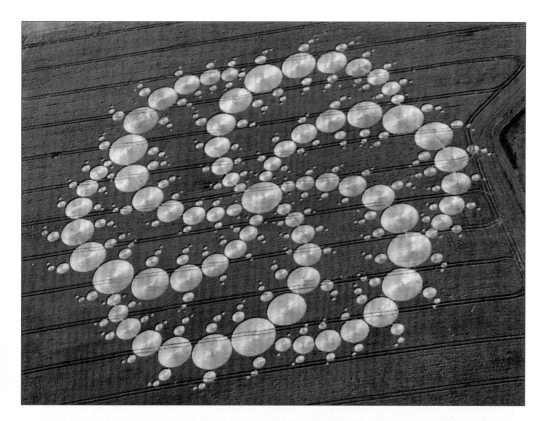

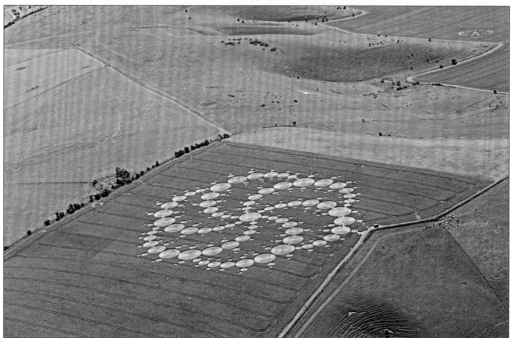

Figs. 6.4 and 6.5. Milk Hill, Alton Barnes, Wiltshire, August 14, 2001 (The Jaw Dropper). A very impressive six armed Julia set design, which spans over ten tramlines.

it also worked perfectly. It is now eleven days later, and the big battery is still charged and the camera working perfectly.

THE JAW DROPPER

As a final note to this formation I include a message I received from the Circle Makers, John Lunberg, Rod Dickinson and Will Russell, who aptly christened the formation the "Jaw Dropper."

> Here's something to ponder. If this formation was man made, allowing for time to get into and out of the field under cover of darkness, the construction time left should be around four hours.
>
> Given that there are over 400 circles, some of which span approx. 70 feet in diameter, that would mean that one of those circles would need to be created every 30 seconds, and that's not even allowing any time for the surveying, purely flattening. This formation pushes the envelope and that's a MASSIVE understatement . . . my brain hurts!

Whereas I do not approve of many of their activities, I was delighted to receive this email and their commendable acknowledgement that the "Jaw Dropper" was beyond the wit of man.

Not only did this formation appear during a rainy night, but on inspection the following day, it revealed no traces of mud on the flattened crop such as would have been clearly visible had people walked down the muddy tramlines to construct it. In addition, the ground was deeply rutted yet the formation showed no jagged edges to the many circles. It lay on the highest point in Wiltshire, the Wansdyke.

MOBILE PHONES

So frequent are mobile-telephone failures that when one fails it comes as no surprise. "I did try my mobile phone in the circle and got a message saying there was no signal, but that wasn't particularly unusual."

On another occasion, on reaching the center of the formation, to my amazement, my switched-off mobile telephone rang in my pocket. I switched it off again and explorer John Blashford Snell, one of the party, said, "Switch it on again and ring the number back." I did as instructed and on the display board it read, "Number unavailable"!

My mobile then (again switched off) started making strange noises, and when I picked it up, it was ringing the same person whom it rang yesterday. I didn't have any numbers in the address book in the phone, so it just picked up a number previously rung.

In contrast, a crop circle visitor recalls that he had used his mobile phone the previous Friday at which time it registered half full; on leaving the crop circle formation it was fully charged!

In the 080808 Alton Barnes formation a visitor using her mobile telephone on entering the formation found that it cut out inside the circle but worked perfectly on leaving.

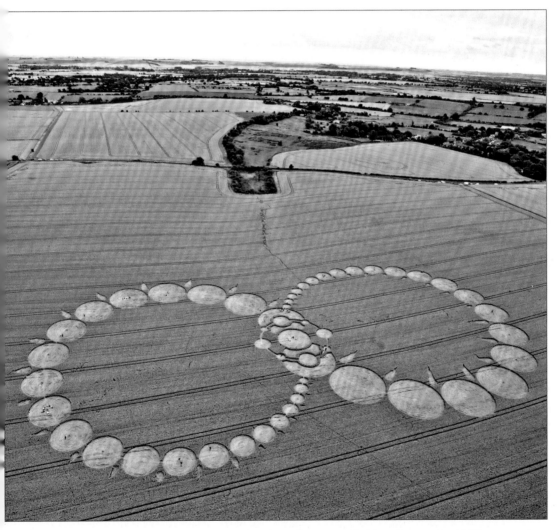

Fig. 6.6. 080808, below Milk Hill, Alton Barnes, Wiltshire, August 8, 2008.

I'm afraid the Sugar Hill formation has been the death knell of my idio-syncratic mobile! Visited the formation late yesterday morning (August 4). Wanted to ring a friend to say it was worth a visit, but could only get a min-imal signal—took phone down tramline, and no signal at all, so decided it was because the field was in a dip. But the signal has never returned—tried in various places all the way home; once got a message on the screen saying "Access Denied" but apart from that nothing. Battery OK, just no signal. Boosted battery when I got back, but nothing doing! Will take mobile into the shop sometime and see what they say, and will let you know.

An addendum from three days later:

Quite extraordinary—switched the mobile on several times yesterday to check for signal. Nothing. Same again this morning. Met friend for lunch and was telling her the story of its demise, switched it on, and suddenly a faint signal, but didn't last long enough to make a call. Same again ten minutes later. But half an hour later, full signal and full service resumed. So it had been out of action for about forty-eight hours, and now seems back to normal—though whether normal is normal or its own version remains to be seen!

CREDIT CARDS AND KEYS

In 1999, after leaving the Hackpen formation, Christopher Weeks discovered that the three bank and credit cards he had brought with him into the forma-tion no longer worked. They had been wiped clean. This would indicate the presence of an oscillating electromagnetic field or, according to Rodney Hale, even a simple direct current (DC) field would achieve this result, which is why we should not place our credit cards near fridge magnets.

Christopher Bean and his friend Linda also had problems in this circle: "I also noticed that my credit cards and bank cards now do not work after taking my wallet into that formation. I only take a few credit cards and bank cards with me when I go out with Linda to the fields so that I can travel light; in this case the ones I'd left behind are fine, but I have had new cards from Royal Bank of Scotland and Barclays (and I am waiting for a new MBNA card)."

Boots, the pharmacy, has a warning sign reminding customers not to put

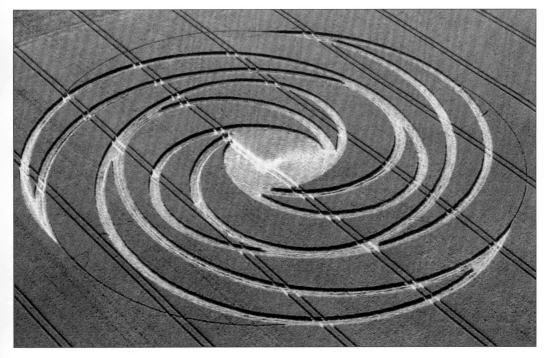

Fig. 6.7. Hackpen, near Broad Hinton, Wiltshire, July 3, 1999.

their debit or credit cards near a certain area of the cash register as the magnetic field can damage them.

James Lyons suggests that for this to happen the electromagnetic field would be turbulent and oscillating at approximately 1,000 cycles per second.

A visitor from abroad found that after visiting the 070707 formation (fig. 6.8, page 92) in East Field, Alton Barnes, the hotel card to her room had also been wiped clean.

A woman who took her remote keyless car-entry device into this same East Field formation (070707) found, on her return to her car, that her device had been completely wiped, and it was now unusable! The information can be erased or reset when exposed to strong ultraviolet light of a certain wavelength, whilst the flash RAM can be cleared or scrambled with an electrical charge. The controller chip would need a significant electrical charge to disrupt operations, along the lines of an electromagnetic pulse (EMP).

Another report came from Sally Ann Mudge who, after visiting a circle, felt very disoriented and even tried to get into the wrong car. When the keys did not fit she thought the formation had interfered with her keys before she realized her error. She felt completely disoriented and feared for her sanity.

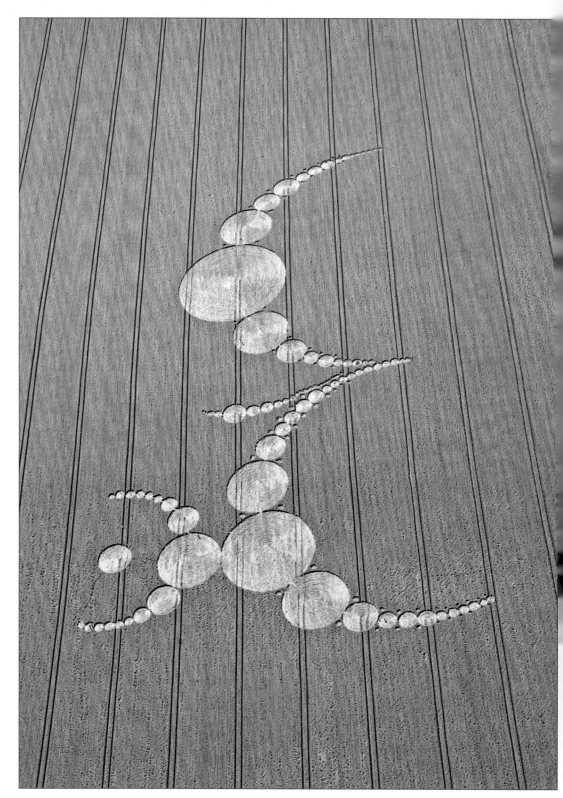

Fig. 6.8. 070707, East Field, Alton Barnes, Wiltshire, July 7, 2007.

On another occasion, Henrik Lovdokken and his wife joined me for a private-entry visit to Stonehenge. He reported:

> However, coming back to our hotel, both of our credit-card-size magnetic hotel keys did not work. It looks like they had been exposed to some magnetic fields from the crop circle visits, causing them to be demagnetized. Demagnetization could happen if it is near a cell phone, but mine was in my wallet all the time and my wife did not carry a cell phone.

CHURCH BELLS

On the night the Double Helix circle appeared (June 17, 1996) in East Field, Alton Barnes, shortly before midnight, a couple living close by heard church bells ringing from the direction of Avebury. They made enquiries and were told the bells were not rung on Sundays and certainly not at midnight. They met an old woman in Avebury who had also heard them ringing that night.

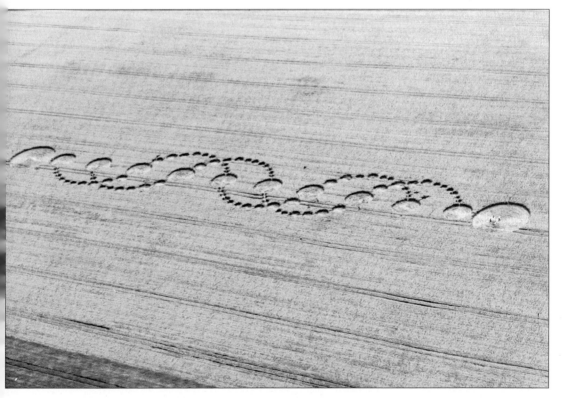

Fig. 6.9. Double Helix, East Field, Alton Barnes, Wiltshire, June 17, 1996.

The bells are not electronically operated; they are rung mechanically. We know that the electromagnetic field caused by UFOs can cause electrical disturbances, but how were the bells mechanically activated on that night of the New Moon in June?

Heather, another visitor, later went into Devizes and was surprised that her pedometer had registered a higher distance walked than expected. "Then I realized that it had altered itself to kilometers. This could not have been done accidentally as one has to hold down the button firmly for five seconds to alter settings."

COMPUTER

During our scientific research day at the Druids' Knot formation (fig. 6.3, page 85) in 2002, Dr. Roger Taylor was anxious about the safety of his laptop computer (owing to the numerous electrical failures that have occurred over the years inside crop circles). He wanted to monitor voltage pulses while inside the formation, so he took his computer in. With him was chartered electrical engineer Rodney Hale, who had adapted a Psion 3A handheld computer to record and graph the rates of any voltages pulses.

All was quiet until 1620 hours (4:20 pm) and then a few minutes later a spike occurred, lasting approximately six minutes (see fig. 6.10).

I telephoned Taylor the next day to inquire about the results and was astounded to learn that since leaving the formation his laptop computer had become useless to the point that it would be necessary to replace the system

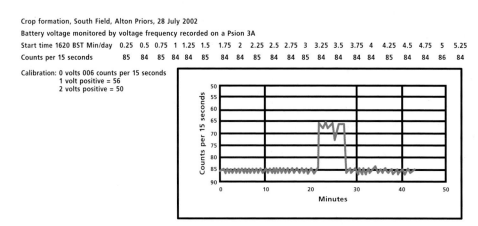

Crop formation, South Field, Alton Priors, 28 July 2002

Battery voltage monitored by voltage frequency recorded on a Psion 3A

Start time 1620 BST Min/day	0.25	0.5	0.75	1	1.25	1.5	1.75	2	2.25	2.5	2.75	3	3.25	3.5	3.75	4	4.25	4.5	4.75	5	5.25
Counts per 15 seconds	85	84	85	84	84	85	84	84	85	84	84	85	84	84	84	84	85	84	84	86	84

Calibration: 0 volts 006 counts per 15 seconds
1 volt positive = 56
2 volts positive = 50

Fig. 6.10. A spike in voltage recorded at the Druids' Knot,
July 28, 2002.

board. Would the results still be there on the hard disk when repaired? Could the six-minute spike recorded on Rodney Hale's Psion handheld computer be held responsible for the damage? Several weeks later, and at a cost of £610 ($800), the computer was restored and yes, his results were still there.

So what could be the cause of the anomalies? Clearly the exact location on the Earth's grid-line pattern—essential for the formation of crop circles—is important, as many areas are especially electrically active. Crossover points of energy lines generate columnar vortices, which are rising spiraling columns of electrical charge. This is a natural consequence of the strong electrostatic potential associated with the Earth-ionosphere electric field. In recent years, equipment capable of measuring these effects has become available.

One word of warning I believe is important. If people have an electrical health device, such as a pacemaker, I would advise them not to enter a crop circle unless they have consulted their doctor.

COMMENTS BY JAMES LYONS

Why do crop circles have such a wide range of effects on so many different items of electrical equipment?

The energy of crop circles is spiraling electric charge. In this respect the energy spirals like a tornado, which reveals its electric origin as filamentary structures rising vertically. This is the basis of crop circle generation. In addition, within crop circles, there are far narrower yet similar structures emerging from the Earth's grid-line structures at nodal points. We measure these with special electrostatic meters.

However, if a laptop, for example, were to be located on such a spot, it would encounter a rotational electric field, which generates magnetic patterns on appropriate structures such as computer-processing electronics. These can often lead to totally scrambled signal structures, which clearly can, at a minimum, distort information but often can so disturb results as to be useless. It is almost impossible to anticipate such effects. The initial testing for such locations permits avoidance of such places. These effects often result in headaches for observers in these places.

There are many investigators of such phenomena. In the early days of the current outbreak of the crop circle phenomenon, many American visitors used standard electrical-energy recording devices with dramatically differing results.

However, research colleagues from Russia are well versed in subtle-energy research and utilized quite specific test equipment. The whole topic of the subtle-energy domain is within mainstream physics, and as such the crop circle scenario is of great interest. In contrast to this more scientific approach, there are many visitors who generally possess, quite naturally, a sensitive response to these rather uniquely structured fields of energy. They represent the majority of crop circle visitors.

The future of the crop circle phenomenon is likely to grow significantly, since interest in the topic of an Electrical Universe is growing dramatically. Generally speaking, gravity is no longer thought to be the key organizing feature in cosmology. Rather electricity, seen as propagated in spiral filaments, is rising to prominence as an important factor. The dramatic changes within our own Solar System, even within the period of recorded history, are at long last being recognized. Archaeological sites such as the Bosnian Pyramid of the Sun with its man-made tunnels have been dated by the British Museum to 34,000 years BCE. The now-recorded columnar vortices rising from its peak resemble the structure of many crop circles. All told, the coherence of many apparently differing phenomena on Earth have a common underlying energy structure. This is leading to a new perspective of the Cosmos and our place within it.

We can now say bye-bye to Big Bang and its offspring, Dark Energy and Dark Matter. Such bizarre concepts are being replaced by evidence for the Electrical Universe. It is not without significance that the crop circle phenomenon has made, and continues to make, a contribution to this world-changing perspective about the Cosmos. We are at last uniting ancient and modern science with life in general, and mankind in particular is playing a significant role in this whole remarkable process.

7

ANIMAL REACTIONS

You have noticed that everything an Indian does is in a circle, and that is because the Power of the World always works in circles, and everything tries to be round. . . . The Sky is round, and I have heard that the Earth is round like a ball, and so are all the stars. The wind, in its greatest power, whirls. Birds make their nest in circles, for theirs is the same religion as ours. . . . Even the seasons form a great circle in their changing, and always come back again to where they were. The life of a man is a circle from childhood to childhood, and so it is in everything where power moves.

BLACK ELK (OGLALA) (1863–1950)

NO MATTER HOW DISMISSIVE SKEPTICS may be about the volume of human and electrical anomalies, animal reactions and behavior are more difficult if not impossible to ignore, and so their behavior is critical to research into crop circles.

We know from the effects on pilots' instruments that there is a vertical field of "energy" that extends to an unknown height above a crop circle; therefore it comes as no surprise that birds are affected. "Whilst sitting enjoying the food and the view of the stones of Avebury, a wood pigeon flew across the field from an easterly direction. Just outside the formation it seemed to almost hit a wall, making it veer suddenly, around the formation, to the north (it didn't overfly it at all) and then it continued to fly to the west after its detour."

Exactly the same effect was recorded in Canada when a skein of geese veered sharply away from flying over a formation, only to regroup directly afterward and continue on their way. Birds have magnetite in their brains and react to magnetic fields.

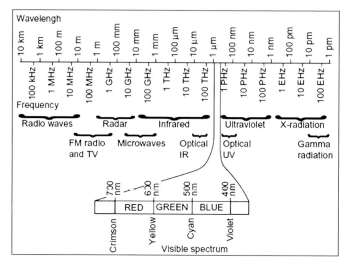

Fig. 7.1. Electromagnetic spectrum.

More sinister were the remains of exploded birds found in the Wanborough crop circle in July 1994. On careful examination it seemed that a bird had exploded in the center of the circle. Christopher Weeks and I found an area measuring in a thirteen- to fourteen-foot radius from the center, covered in blood, tiny feathers, and minute bits of flesh, not just on the surface but penetrating every layer right to ground level. There were no bones or any distinguishable parts of the bird, and the "mess" was totally different in appearance from the pile of feathers in the outer ring, clearly once belonging to a pigeon and clearly killed by a fox. We sent samples to a biologist in Devon who reported that indeed it would appear that a bird had "exploded" and that it was dead at the time of the explosion. I had found empty cartridge cases in the field, and it was clear that the pigeon had been shot and was lying there and had disintegrated when the crop circle force hit the ground.

Another report on the darker side spoke of

the strangest and most chilling thing I have ever seen was the body of a hedgehog which appeared to have been completely drained of body fluids— as if it had been freeze-dried. I grew up in the country, so have seen lots of dead wildlife, but never have I seen anything like this. It was on the path

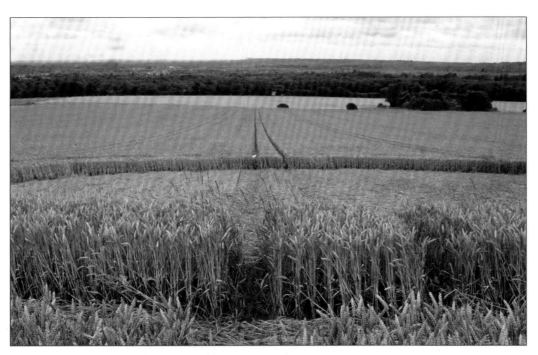

Fig. 7.2. Wanborough, near Guildford, Surrey, July 1994.

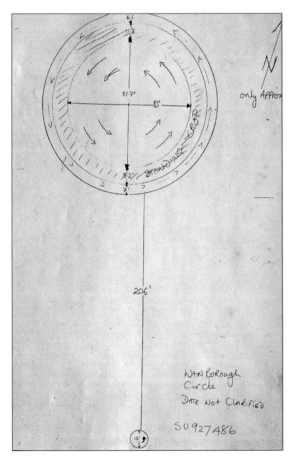

Fig. 7.3. Wanborough, near Guildford, Surrey.

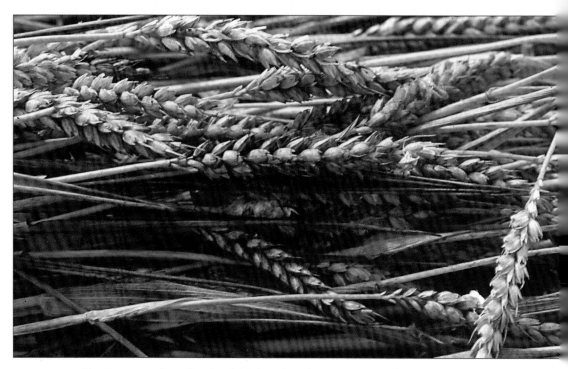

Fig. 7.4. Remains of a dead bird within the Wanborough circle, July 1994.

into the formation at Avebury Trusloe, June/July 1991. There appeared to be no external injuries, but it looked almost flat.

The friend who was with me at the time was used to picking up roadkill for a friend of his who is a taxidermist, but he had seen nothing like this. I would have taken it away but my friend was adamant that it was not going in his car!

This report is similar to the dehydrated and flattened porcupines that were found in a crop circle in Canada in 1992. The dehydrated corpses showed no signs of injury or decomposition and did not smell. Animals can sense danger, but both hedgehogs and porcupines rely on their quills to protect them and therefore remain stationary instead of fleeing. In these cases we seem to be dealing with the microwave, infrared area of the electromagnetic spectrum, suggesting that these animals were indeed "microwaved."

CHARACTER CHANGE

Some normally docile creatures seem to behave in uncharacteristic ways when exposed to samples of crops from the formations. Doreen Jenkinson had taken home some wheat from inside a newly formed crop circle, and as soon as she got home her customarily sweet and gentle cat started growling at her in a low tone as Doreen touched the wheat. "I normally hang the wheat up but because of my cat's reaction I left it in the lavatory. My cat sat 'guarding' it for two days. After one day I went to touch the wheat and got the same reaction from her, glaring at me to say 'No, don't touch.' By the second day this reaction disappeared."

My gray cat, Hero, became obsessed with some stalks of barley from a crop event that I put under the dining room table. He sat there sucking the ears of the barley and growled at me when I tried to remove him. He would sit by the dining room door, dashing in to resume the "sucking" each time I opened the door. I also noticed that his character was changing, and he was becoming aggressive. He was a beautiful big gray cat, and I loved him so much.

Alarm bells started ringing, however, when one time I went into the dining room for something and refused to let him in. I bent down to stroke him as I came out and he suddenly stood up on his hind legs and almost raked my face with his claws. I realized that something was desperately wrong, and despite all treatments, including homeopathic remedies, his day-to-day aggression increased to the point that he became a serious danger to me, and sadly I had to have him put down, which nearly broke my heart.

It all started after he sucked the barley stalks. Had there been some chemical reaction from sucking the stalks? Was it due to various crop sprays used by the farmers?

HE IS THE CAT'S WHISKERS

In early July, I took a party of people from London into the bewitchingly beautiful South Field "Cathedral" formation.

I had given them a talk in the morning, and before I started was surprised to be greeted by a stranger, accompanied by a cat in a British Airways bag slung over her shoulder. The woman asked after my cat, Hero. How did she know about Hero? Of course, I had mentioned him in my book, and Rupert, the Burmese blue, was here to experience the circles for himself.

It was one of those days when every type of weather condition was practicing its skills with the greatest of enthusiasm and gusto. One moment, the Sun would peek its nose through briefly only to be shouldered out by the clouds, the bringers of rain—rain of every sort and description from a drizzle to torrential downpours accompanied by thunder and lightning. It seemed that we had to experience the whole bacchanalian menu of conditions. How were these townies going to survive this wanton display by the elements? They were magnificent: many of them had never been into a crop formation before, and many of them were strangers to the countryside. For them the whole scenario turned into a magical, mystical event as we stood in the formation surrounded by the ancient hills terraced by our ancestors of long ago, the nipple on the breast of Adam's Grave standing out proudly, reminding us of our connection with Gaia.

What about Rupert? If an animal could talk then surely he would be the first; he was a most sagacious beast and apparently accompanied his owner

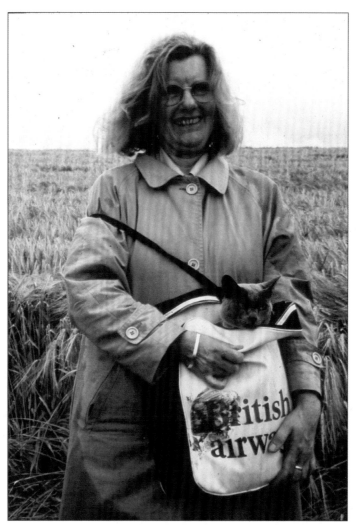

Fig. 7.5. Mary Spain and Rupert the cat, 2000.

nearly everywhere. He was attached to a very long leather lead giving him maximum independence. His owner Mary Spain writes:

> The most interesting aspect of Rupert's reactions was that he behaved exactly as he does when visiting a church—he has visited numerous country churches on our travels. He was respectful, quiet, alert, and very interested. When on a country walk he is far more boisterous. Another interesting thing was that, uninvited, he went up to a stranger sitting meditating and sat down beside her. Although he is always perfectly polite to strangers, he is not normally friendly to this extent and has never sat on anyone's lap but mine.
>
> It may be coincidence, but Rupert's constipation problems were sorted out after the experience!

An intriguing end to this story came to my notice. Mary Spain wrote telling me that five days after visiting the formation, she went to have her hair cut.

> My hairdresser couldn't understand the amount of static in my hair until I explained that it had been full of energy since I visited a crop circle at the weekend. She grew very excited saying that only that morning she had seen a beautiful picture of a crop circle in the *Daily Mail* and had read of Rupert's experiences.

HORSE SENSE

A beautiful Daisy Chain formation in barley was discovered at Cheriton, near Cheesefoot Head, Hampshire, on July 6, 1997. The surrounding twenty-nine circles around the flattened center each contained a central tuft of standing crop; diagonally across the center of the formation were two "Magimix blades" consisting of minute and perfect circles.

An American researcher was the first to discover and visit the formation. She had neglected to ask the farmer's permission and, as she was standing in the circle, the farmer's wife came riding down the tramlines toward her. As the woman got nearer she rode toward the unfortunate researcher in an aggressive manner, but the moment her horse reached the edge of the circle it stopped, and despite several cracks of the whip, refused to budge, becoming quite agitated. This clearly added to the rider's annoyance, and she shouted, "I do not believe in these %#@& circles!"

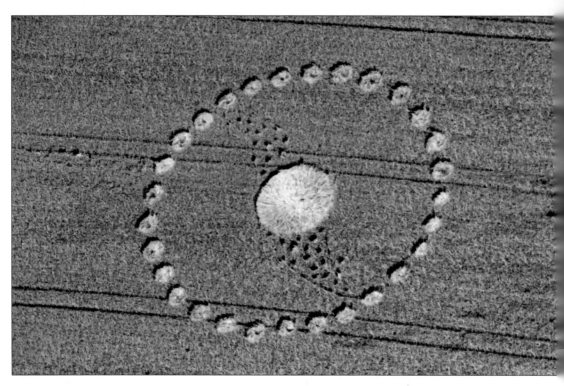

Fig. 7.6. Daisy Chain at Cheriton,
near Cheesefoot Head, Hampshire, July 4, 1997.

"Maybe you don't, but your horse certainly does!" replied the researcher.

In that year, one of my first visits was to the "Bear's Paw" near Morested, Hampshire, which appeared in early May in barley. A rider was trotting her gray horse along the path dividing the field in two. I managed to catch her before she disappeared out of sight and asked her if she would mind riding her horse into the formation.

She was happy to do so, saying she was fascinated by the crop circles and had taken her horse into several. She felt he was a good judge of the circle's authenticity. Her horse displayed no visible sign of agitation, moving around the formation and standing still when reined in. The rider however remarked that his breathing rate had noticeably increased.

What made a Rottweiler rushing ahead of its owner into a crop circle suddenly stop dead, roll over, and fall asleep just before it reached a terrified woman sitting meditating in the center?

Equally strange was the behavior of two normally friendly Labradors, as shown when they attacked each other and then a woman inside a formation.

What conclusion can we reach, if any? Can we ascribe this varied and bizarre behavior to certain frequencies in the electromagnetic field, or could we be dealing with the effects of crop spraying?

I suspect that the young wheat in that field had already had a potent mix of a whole range of herbicides, insecticides, and fungicides sprayed upon it, with a lot more to go.

I really feel that people should look on the website of various organizations to find out more about these symptoms. I know there is a couple working at the University of Iowa on agricultural chemical poisoning. We should remember that most spray applications are what are called "tank mixes" where, to save time and money, farmers mix several sprays at once, often up to four different brands. This can cause a little-understood range of chemical interactions.

I am now beginning to believe that many of the experiences people record within these fields are directly related to chemical poisoning, and anyone going into a field would be well advised to check with the farmer what his spraying regime had been. I know that, speaking personally, I will not be entering another circle unless I have first checked with the farmer about when the field was last sprayed.

COMMENTS BY JAMES LYONS

So far, our consideration of ambient energy within crop circles has, not surprisingly, focused on humans. However, as we have already observed, we must at least consider the circles' interaction with other living species.

Here we'll focus on two creatures: dogs, who on many occasions have accompanied their owners into crop circles, and birds, which, of course, are more likely to overfly formations and yet are still susceptible to the specific ambient energy fields.

Since these creatures possess similar consciousness-related cell structures as humans, we need to assess what similarities and differences relate to behavior. As with all living creatures, it is the structure of the brain that mainly accounts for the observed effects. With regard to humans, we need to consider brain frequency and energy-detection processes. Concentrating on the latter, which has so far received little attention, there is one common feature, including among humans, which can be clearly identified as the key element of energy detection.

We assume that the eyes are the major information-detection system, but sight clearly depends on light waves within a relatively narrow frequency spectrum, namely, the colors of the rainbow. Yet a completely separate system is needed to detect and process information when we consider the ambient waves within a crop circle. These waves are the spiraling waves of electric charge, which dominate the structure of the Cosmos.

We mentioned above that these are called torsion waves, as per our Slinky model; these waves can be detected by what in early Yogic philosophy was called the Third Eye, which is connected to the pineal gland, so called because of its pinecone-shaped structure. The gland is in essence made of quartz and hence is, as all Healers know, electrically active.

It operates in a completely different way from the eyes, which use frequencies far higher than the fundamental resonance frequency of quartz. The frequency of quartz is 28 kHz, a little above the hearing limit of humans. This frequency has recently been identified in the columnar vortex rising from the Bosnian Pyramid of the Sun. It is also the frequency used in low-voltage health zappers that interact at the cellular level. The third eye is the detector of all the spiraling waves we find in not only crop circles but all ancient sites.

Dogs have a higher frequency-response range than humans and are aware of the Earth vibrations. Depending on the spectrum of these frequencies, a dog will behave in differing ways. As young people devour the frequencies of rock music, older folk mostly prefer Vivaldi!

It is the bird scenario that is perhaps even more fascinating. For around 150 years, people have thought that birds navigate by detecting the Earth's magnetic field, especially magnetic north. To date, despite enormous effort, no one has found any sign of such a feature that could possibly be used for navigation.

However, a completely new model is emerging based on the use of the pineal gland as the key detector of the key frequency of the Earth, which is identifiable at many locations on our planet. Like the Bosnian pyramid and crop circles, as well as ancient sites and medieval churches, there is a columnar vortex of energy generated at points on the Earth's energy grid that provides an enormous directional signal like a lighthouse.

There have been many situations in which flocks of birds flying toward ancient sites or crop circles split into two groups, each flying around the column and joining up again once past it. They have no problem detecting the spiraling energy via their pineal systems. Work continues on how pineal glands link via the hypothalamus to the brain to reveal and analyze the emitted columnar vortex—the perfect navigation system.

Additionally, a pineal gland can act like an accelerometer as well as a rate gyro, the two key building blocks of an inertial navigation system. Perhaps the most revealing aspect of this new hypothesis is that the subtle energy field around the pineal gland reduces sharply to zero when its axis is pointing at magnetic north.

Thus we see that crop circle energies, created initially by rising toroidal waveforms that rise from underground water, when breaking through the Earth's surface, form a vacuum space to draw down the crop. This leaves a spiraling columnar vortex in which we find a whole spectrum of frequencies, mostly within the frequency band compatible with the detection systems of humans, animals, and birds. It is therefore of no surprise that reactions to these signals are perfectly normal. The frequencies involved can generate both good and bad responses, dependent on the health condition of the human or animal.

To conclude this section, it is worth noting that it is at long last possible to purchase Radionic Healing units. These are quite old in concept, but computerized equipment now enables such units, via handheld probes, to analyze the frequency response of a complete patient.

As an orchestral conductor tunes up his players prior to a concert, modern radionics units analyze each organ of the body, for example, the heart or lungs, to see how out of tune a patient is. With such a "map" it becomes possible to retune that organ to its correct operating frequency. No pharmaceuticals are needed. Such units are now being evaluated in the NHS, and large-scale implementation of the technology is envisaged.

8

SCIENTIFIC
AND MEDICAL TESTING

Time comes from the future, which does not yet exist, into the present, which has no duration, and goes into the past, which has ceased to exist.

SAINT AUGUSTINE (354–430)

AS I NOTED IN THE PROLOGUE, after my own personal healing experience in 1990, I realized that there must be many other people experiencing similar effects, and, in order to try and explore what was happening, I drew up a rudimentary first questionnaire to give to those visiting crop circles. I was amazed by the huge response.

Little did I realize what a wealth of material I would accumulate over the years as a result of that remarkable day in July 1990, and I now have the largest database in the world relating to crop circle effects with an impressive collection of over eight hundred reports. These were not reports of random experiences; there were too many strange and varied personal events to ignore.

I am of the opinion that we are, as indeed are all living things, composed of "energies." These energies ebb and flow depending on a number of things, for example, our emotional and physical well-being. These energies extend to varying degrees *beyond* our actual *physical* bodies. I wonder how many of you understand why you react the way you do if you are in close proximity to another person? Your energy fields (or aura) are in fact overlapping, and you will find that you are on the same wavelength (vibrations or energies) as that person, to a greater or lesser degree, having the possibility of varying from one extreme to the other. Hence you may register abhorrence, dislike, being vaguely uneasy, neutrality—right through to total compatibility.

How often we put on a façade in order to appear as we *think* others would like to see us; we are all chameleons, and in order to survive and adapt we so often disguise our true self. However, from those who can feel or see the energy force there can be no concealment. They will be able to know intuitively the physical and emotional well-being of each individual. So it is with all living things; even leather and wood breathe. The Earth is a mighty energy force of a complexity not comprehended by many. For the Earth's responses are controlled by many interacting and interdependent conditions, among them the other planetary influences being forces of great importance. Remember, the planet is a living, breathing organism, which we with great temerity would try and harness for our own greedy benefit.

Now for the crop circle energies: where these involve ley lines, and indeed it would seem that this is the case with all (apart from the hoaxed ones), the energies present are powerful. Thus the reactions of individuals will relate to their own personal energies. Some may be unpleasant, others extremely harmonious and beneficial. In all events it is a *very personal* experience, and I have seen a number of people come quietly out of a circle with a look of awe and humility: a far cry from the persons they were when they went in! It is also important to point out that should you feel in any way uncomfortable, you should leave as quickly as possible. There is no point in persisting, and indeed it could be harmful. Experiences have varied from healing to headaches!

Whereas the skeptical may, with a certain amount of justification, dismiss out of hand the results of the human-effects reports as coming from people with overactive imaginations, it is more difficult to dismiss the evidence of rigorously conducted scientific tests. To be fair, I cannot dismiss the number of reports I have received from people who have taken the trouble to fill in and return the questionnaires. I believe the majority are sober-minded, levelheaded people. I realize it can be a time-consuming and lengthy procedure filling out forms, but they are of the utmost importance, and are written with such amazing descriptive clarity and vividness, as if the contributors have painted a picture with words. There can be absolutely no doubt that these experiences were real, and people's sincerity and amazement at what had happened to them were beyond any reasonable question. Indeed I know from my own personal experience that there are many varied "energies" in the circles that can affect people individually.

Once you have had a personal experience there is absolutely no doubt in your mind that something out of the ordinary has happened to you for which you can find no other logical explanation no matter how hard you try.

THE PLACEBO EFFECT

At this point I must make clear that it has been suggested that a placebo effect could be involved in the healing process of people visiting the crop circles or indeed watching them on screen. This is a perfectly valid assumption and one that needs to be addressed.

What is a placebo effect? Used medically, it is a process of testing the effectiveness of a treatment in which a proportion of the people being tested are given the actual medical treatment and the rest are given a visually identical treatment but one that is designed to have no effect over a given length of time. If some of the people who are not given the real medical treatment feel better, this is put down to the placebo effect.

When people visit a crop circle the general presumption is that they are going to feel well or even feel better as a result. If we look at the other side of the coin, you will be surprised to find that this is frequently not the case and defies all their strongly held expectations. Considering that I have a database of over eight hundred reports, it seems unlikely that so many people could all be suffering from delusion or overactive imaginations when sometimes they have experienced really quite intense disagreeable effects, as well as beneficial ones on other occasions. It is interesting to note the amazement and bewilderment experienced by people to these contrary and unpleasant effects. Many regular visitors now realize that the effects of visiting a crop circle cannot be prejudged, as the effects are felt on such an individual basis; one person might be sitting in a crop circle feeling wonderful, whereas the person sitting beside them feels ill. This seems to be dependent on the many aspects involved in the mental, physical, and emotional well-being of each person.

The same reactions may be found with only visual exposure. Photographs shown in a book or on the screen are emitting frequencies with the same negative results, some of which are so extreme to the point that some people have had to leave the slide lecture or stop reading the book because they have felt so ill. On the flip side, ailments and illnesses can be healed. Again, I stress that we are dealing with individuals, and so the effects will of necessity be varied and multiple.

It has also been proposed that "suggestion" could play a large part in any scientific test, that being wired up with electrodes plus the expectation of benefit and so forth could indeed induce people to believe that they will "feel" better. Therefore it is particularly interesting to note that there was one interesting set of scientific research conducted at Avebury Trusloe near Windmill Hill, Wiltshire, in 2006. We were particularly excited as the circle had appeared that very morning and so was fresh. However, the results were disappointing, with little or no apparent change between the control tests taken at Avebury, near Marlborough, Wiltshire, and identical tests taken inside the newly formed crop circle. I was later reliably informed that this circle had been man made. We had indeed unintentionally conducted a most useful and instructive set of double-blind tests.

THE MEMORY OF WATER

Back to people's reports of their experiences in crop circles: What are these "energies" that they describe? With so many reports coming in, clearly I needed to try and find an answer to what these energies were and what was happening to people who experienced them.

I am on a tremendous learning curve, investigating areas not previously studied. This could only be regarded as enormously exciting; not only in scientific terms but in making me aware that there is an ocean of knowledge and wisdom still eluding us. This knowledge is inherent in Nature itself, and it is to Nature, at its most profound and spiritual level, that we needed to look for the answers.

My first idea (much to the derision of my peers!) was to bury small bottles of water inside a crop circle and compare them with bottles of water taken from the same source but buried outside the circle. I had long held the belief that, as water possessed unique qualities, if anything might possibly register a measureable change when in contact within a crop circle, as opposed to outside, it would be water. These have been analyzed over the years using different techniques, and the results have been quite remarkable. Water has a unique quality to it, and despite great strides in medicine, physics, chemistry, and biology, water and its behavior still remains largely a mystery. I believed that if anything was going to reveal what was happening in the crop circles, it would be water.

We are told (in an article by Robert Matthews) that whereas most substances are denser in their solid form than when they are liquid, water is less dense. Most substances shrink when cool, yet frozen water expands, taking up more space than the original liquid.

The boiling point, melting point, and heat-conducting abilities of water are far higher than other substances, and it takes more energy to boil a pint of water than any other liquid.

An average adult body is 50 to 60 percent water; that is roughly equivalent to 45 quarts. Men are more watery than women. A man's body is 60 to 65 percent water, compared to 50 to 60 percent for a woman. In infants, the figure is a whopping 70 percent, according to statistics compiled by the International Bottled Water Association.

About 70 percent of the Earth's surface is covered in water, and the oceans hold about 97 percent of all the Earth's water yet more that 95 percent of the underwater world remains unexplored. But water also exists in the air as vapor, in rivers and lakes, and in icecaps and glaciers.

Over a period of many years, the bottles I buried were sent to many laboratories and were tested using different techniques. The results of the tests were astounding, not only in their consistency but in the way the water responded to being buried inside the circles as compared to the control samples outside. Since 1992 I have been burying bottles of water in crop circles using the following procedure. Following Dr. Cyril Smith's advice, I used Volvic water as being the most constant water, not going above 4 Hz. Control samples are buried first outside the formation and the others inside. When collecting the bottles, the ones inside are collected first and the control samples second, in order that the control samples are never influenced by the "energies" inside the circle. I carry a notebook with me to give me an indication of where the bottles have been buried, but as many people often trample the circle, the basic ground lay of the fallen crop may have altered the result so we turn to dowsing in order to find and retrieve the bottles. Over many years we have found over 95 percent. The bottles are labeled and numbered and written up in my notebook as I bury them, then wrapped in silver kitchen paper, placed in an egg box, and sent to a laboratory to be tested blind. I am the only person who knows which number relates to each bottle and its buried whereabouts.

In the July 2010 Vernham Dean formation the following water results were of interest. Christopher Weeks and I buried bottles of Volvic water inside the circle in different areas. The further out toward the edge the worse I felt and eventually said "I have got to get out." My head ached, I felt nauseous, disoriented, and generally drained. However we both managed to bury the one remaining bottle before hurriedly making our exit. We had buried the control samples at the edge of the field before entering the formation, thereby insuring they didn't come into contact with any of the formation "energics."

On retrieving the bottles some ten days later we experienced none of these symptoms. This is something to which we have become accustomed, as the more people visit a circle, the more they seem to soak up and absorb the "residual" original force.

The controls were bottles 273, 274, double control sample 275. A fascinating factor is that the Yara tests for trace minerals revealed an increase in ammonia. There is no ammonia present in a bottle of Volvic water! What was happening? James Lyons kindly supplied a solution. Ammonia is a compound of nitrogen N and hydrogen H with the formula NH_3.

> The first thing to notice is the correlation between the nitrate and ammonia results. It seems as there is some breakdown of water into its constituent parts, namely hydrogen and oxygen. These molecules then attach to free nitrogen atoms creating both increased nitrate NO_3 and ammonia NH_4. This is an interesting finding!

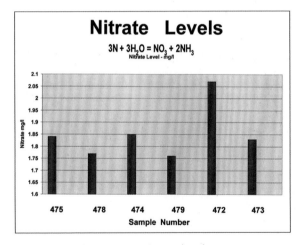

Fig. 8.1. Nitrate levels.

THE PARKINSON'S QUESTION

One remarkable event was the spur to the next area of investigation. It came in a report from a friend of mine, suffering from Parkinson's disease. She desperately wanted to visit a crop circle to see if it could possibly help her. I

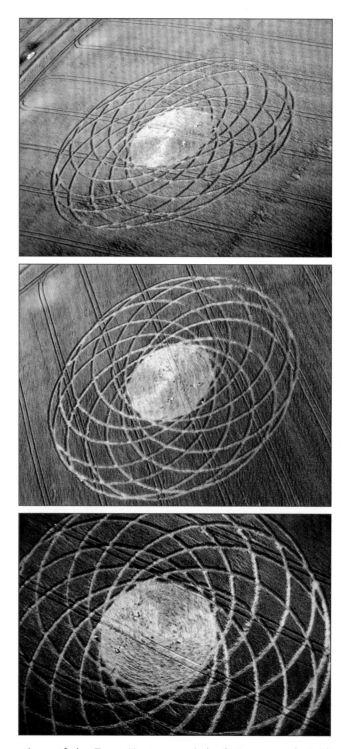

Fig. 8.2. Three views of the Torus Knot crop circle that appeared at Alton Priors, Wiltshire, July 11, 1997.

was reluctant to agree to this in case her condition was exacerbated. However, due to her persistence, I agreed to try and find a circle as nearly 100 percent beneficial as possible. To this end I spent almost a week visiting the "Torus Knot" crop circle that appeared at Alton Priors, Wiltshire, on July 11, 1997. It consisted of a central circle with twelve large interlocking rings around it, similar to a Spirograph pattern, and was approximately 300 feet in diameter. Not only did I go into the circle many times during that week but I also stood by the edge of the field in order to talk to the people as they came out and thus collected many reports, all of which were beneficial. Could this be the circle for my friend? I insisted that it had to be entirely at her own risk and responsibility. A few days later she entered the circle with a friend and experienced a temporary but wonderful physical respite from the exhausting and continuous shaking after sitting in the center for about twenty minutes. Subsequently she did not shake for twenty-four hours. The physical relief was enormous during that period, as was the amazing feeling of well-being that went along with the physical respite.

What was the reason for this extraordinary event? Since Parkinson's disease is a result of a chemical imbalance in the brain, clearly this should be where our search should be directed, and thus began a new quest involving research into the activity of the brain and the endocrine system.

As mentioned in chapter 2, page 27, a teasing thought arises when one thinks about consciousness. Is it a part of the brain or an independent entity? It has been suggested that consciousness may not be generated by the brain but rather "transceived" by it*—that is, that consciousness may be a fundamental "nonlocal" property of all dimensions of the Universe, and that rather than being an "epiphenomenon of brain activity," it may instead be that the brain acts as an interface that allows consciousness to manifest "locally" on the material plane. I feel comfortable with this idea.

However, our research was limited not only by the type of tests we could conduct but also by the techniques and methodology available. We have not been able to conduct blood tests on people before they go into a circle, while they are inside the circle, and later as a double control test. This would have enabled us to investigate the strange acid/metallic taste that I and others have experienced when visiting a circle. The taste is so pervasive; one is unable to get rid of it until it suddenly disappears as soon as one leaves the

---

*See www.huffingtonpost.com/deepak-chopra/reply-to-chris-anderson-t_b_3119890.html.

circle. This could indicate a sudden drop in blood-sugar level and a draining of energy.

As noted in chapter 4, page 47, a lady after a talk came up to me and said, "I have got that taste now, and I am not in a crop circle!" She was a diet-maintained diabetic and knew that as soon as her protein ketones were breaking down, she got this taste in her mouth. Could this be what is happening to people when they visit certain formations? This was exciting yet frustrating due to our research constraints.

THE ANNUAL SCIENTIFIC DAYS

As the years went by we continued to get consistent results that demonstrated changes in hormones (endocrine system) and other related areas including EEG (electroencephalogram) tests, but, frustratingly, no real progress was being made that would explain the temporary relief of Parkinson's, and I was on the brink of giving up—that is, until one day in July 2010 when conducting the annual scientific research investigations in a crop circle at Fosbury, near Vernham Dean, lying on the borders of Hampshire and Wiltshire. The circle consisted of a central cube surrounded by angled Russian doll–type squares inside an outer hexagon, and it had appeared just a few days previously.

VERNHAM DEAN 2010

Using the Asyra technique, acclaimed by William Tiller, professor of materials science and engineering at Stanford University, as one of the most reliable diagnostic systems available, Hazel Drummond reported:

> This year I carried out a test especially for the crop-circle research day. It tested for disturbances/imbalances in the endocrine system, neurotransmitters, brain-wave patterns, chakras, vertebral misalignments, electrolyte disturbances, geopathic stress, harmful energies, and meridian disturbance.
>
> The baseline test, which covers all of the main organs/systems, was also run.
>
> In the results we are primarily looking for patterns of results that are out of the ordinary. For instance, in a standard group of eleven people being tested for any particular disturbance we may well see two or maybe three showing a similar disturbance, but usually it would be none or maybe one. Therefore more than three is significant. The results are then collated.

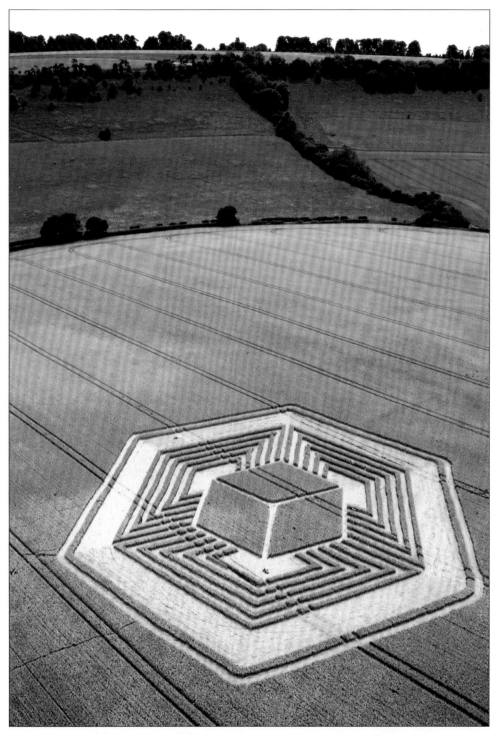

Fig. 8.3. Russian doll–type squares found at the crop circle at
Vernham Dean, Fosbury, Hampshire, July 17, 2010.

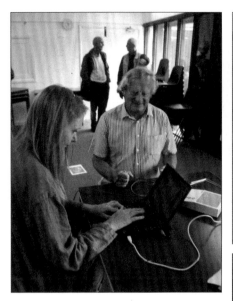

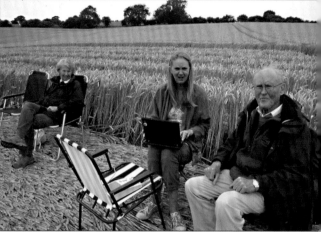

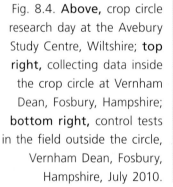

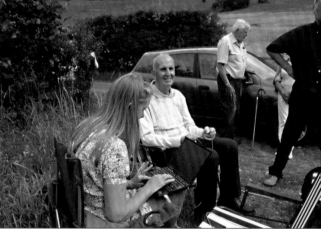

Fig. 8.4. **Above,** crop circle research day at the Avebury Study Centre, Wiltshire; **top right,** collecting data inside the crop circle at Vernham Dean, Fosbury, Hampshire; **bottom right,** control tests in the field outside the circle, Vernham Dean, Fosbury, Hampshire, July 2010.

The first control tests were conducted at the Avebury Study Centre between 10:00 a.m. and midday. For this year's crop-circle research day we had eleven subjects, including myself; there were seven males and four females.

The same tests were then repeated in the crop circle between 2:00 p.m. and 3:00 p.m. Further identical control tests were conducted at the edge of the field bordering the lane after visiting the circle.

I was then able to compare the results to see if there were any significant changes in the three sets of results. As well as comparing the three sets of tests I also compared the results from tests of ten random people. This was the first time that we had tested for unusual activity with brain-wave patterns. When this test is usually run we might see that none of the patterns come up as imbalanced, or one or two out of eleven may have a particular brain-wave pattern imbalance. I was quite surprised to see the patterns that emerged, although again I am not sure of what the meaning may be.

Six people in the circle showed gamma-wave activity (a very high frequency between 32–74 Hz per second).

THE MISSING LINK

Could there be a link to Parkinson's disease? After reading copious articles on the internet, I stumbled on a short paragraph in one that said that the brain naturally produces dopamine in the gamma level of brain activity. This was exciting; as it appears that in the higher frequencies of both beta and gamma more dopamine is released. Could this discovery be the longed-for breakthrough after so many years of backbreaking and seemingly unrewarding research that appeared to be getting us nowhere fast?

Dopamine is an important neurotransmitter (messenger) in the brain.

Further research told me that beta is the frequency range between approximately 13 and 30 Hz and gamma is between approximately 31 and 74 Hz (see fig. 8.5 below). Because of the filtering properties of the skull and scalp, gamma rhythms can only be recorded from electrocorticography or possibly with magnetoencephalography. Gamma rhythms are thought to represent binding of different populations of neurons together into a network for the purpose of carrying out a certain cognitive or motor function.

State	Frequency range	State of mind
Delta	0.5Hz - 4Hz	Deep sleep
Theta	4Hz - 8Hz	Drowsiness (also first stage of sleep)
Alpha	8Hz - 14Hz	Relaxed but alert
Beta	14Hz - 32Hz	Highly alert and focused
Gamma	32Hz - 74Hz	

Fig. 8.5. The relationship between frequency ranges and state of mind.

Gamma brain waves are considered the brain's optimal frequency of functioning. They are commonly associated with increased levels of brain functioning. They are also associated with a conscious awareness of reality and increased mental abilities. As mentioned above, gamma brain waves range from the frequency of 38 Hz to 74 Hz per second and have tiny (virtually unnoticcablc) amplitude. Gamma brain waves can be found in virtually every part of the brain. They also serve as a binding mechanism between all parts of the brain and help to improve memory and perception.

Dopamine is classified as a catecholamine (a class of molecules that serve as neurotransmitters and hormones). It is a monoamine (a compound containing nitrogen formed from ammonia by replacement of one or more of the hydrogen atoms by hydrocarbon radicals). Dopamine is a precursor (forerunner) of adrenaline and a closely related molecule, noradrenaline. Dopamine is formed by the decarboxylation (removal of a carboxyl group) from dopa.

Dopa is used in the treatment of Parkinson's disease, which is often thought to be associated with low levels of dopamine in certain areas of the brain.

Could my friend, who stopped shaking for twenty-four hours after sitting in the Torus Knot formation in 1997, have experienced a sudden burst of gamma-level brain activity resulting in a release of dopa? At long last we were starting to make longed-for progress in understanding this elusive phenomenon.

The following year I got in touch with a neuroscientist at Leicester University. He was intrigued by our findings, as he was finding that by increasing the level of brain activity of Parkinson's sufferers to the gamma level, it inhibited their dyskinesia, that is, it stopped their shaking. However, his research was funded by the Welcome Trust, among others, and owing to the adverse press coverage the crop circle phenomenon receives in the United Kingdom, he was unable to work with us in furthering our research. However, to know that we were on the right track was good enough for me, and that at long last the years of struggling to find a possible solution might be starting to bear fruit.

BARBURY CASTLE 2011

The crop circle research day procedure starts at Avebury Study Centre, near Marlborough, Wiltshire, where we conduct the first control tests. We then proceed to the selected crop circle, repeating the tests, and finally we move out of the circle to a point some distance away and conduct the second control test. These tests are then compared and analyzed.

In 2011 we conducted our research in a formation lying below the famous Iron Age hill fort at Barbury Castle in Wroughton, Wiltshire.

David Greenwood wrote the following report:

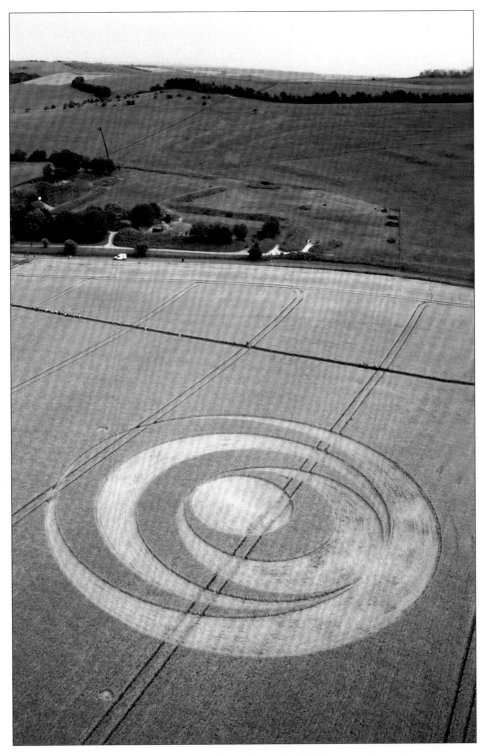

Fig. 8.6. Barbury Castle, Wroughton, Wiltshire, July 2, 2011.

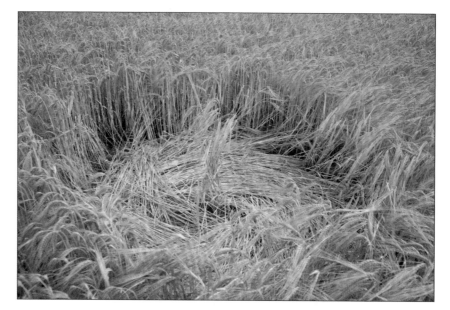

Fig. 8.7. Barbury Castle, Wroughton, Wiltshire, July 2, 2011.

As I approached the crop formation after walking down the track I had the chronic pain in my left lower leg and foot and fatigue, which are the main symptoms that have manifested in me for at least six years now. When I entered the formation I began to walk with the flow of the laid crop and close to the wall of standing crop wondering what intelligence had given the instruction to change from broad to narrow and form the arms of a spiral shape. My awareness of self soon disappeared as I began to enjoy walking the laid path. When I spotted a small depression in the crop I followed the tramline out of the main formation toward the depression. It was at the point when I walked toward the depression that I felt something like a blast of static electricity. It affected my face when both sides of my face felt in compression. The hairs on my neck and arms were prickly. I stopped by the depression and my immediate thought was that it was a nest of some kind. With the stalks crossed in the center I thought it might be a signature or just a sign meant to convey impudence "Work me out! Who am I?" or "I stopped here and left, and this is my tail end." At that point I walked back into the main formation and continued to follow the wall of the crop round until I saw the second and larger nest (satellite). I did not enter this formation because a lady was busy dowsing in the formation. After I had walked the whole of the formation I definitely had a feeling of well-being but noticed that a slight tremor had returned to my left hand. I knelt down in the vortex of the formation and asked my subconscious to tell me the truth—it revealed to me that the formation was astral and a hologram with height and depth meant to convey "As above, so below."

As I left the formation I was quite energized and walking briskly. My attention was drawn to a building called the Science Centre, and I wondered if there might be a connection with the formations. At the end of the visit I was convinced and still am that this formation had been produced by something spinning that produced the static electricity. Certainly it was not a board-and-string formation.

In response to my further questions he kindly replied,

To answer your questions: The tremor stopped after I had entered the crop formation and had walked approximately 30 meters on the laid crop in the direction it had been laid. A slight tremor in my hand returned after I had finished walking the formation.

LIDDINGTON 2012

Since that memorable day in the Vernham Dean formation in 2010 our research has continued with equally exciting and consistent results. Also joining us in 2011 was Paul Gerry, a highly specialized clinical physiologist from the Devon and Exeter Hospital. As the technology improves, so the extent of our research and methodology is widening and expanding each year. Each year we take in volunteer Parkinson's sufferers; also sufferers of Essential Tremor, a condition often linked, but not necessarily so, to Parkinson's disease.

David Greenwood had volunteered to be my Parkinson's guinea pig in 2011 with remarkable results. He had enjoyed the day so much that he re-volunteered to come in 2012. However, at the last moment, his wife fell ill and, as he is unable to drive, he had to abandon joining us.

In 2012, the chosen circle was at Liddington, just off the busy M4 motorway, a complex multidimensional design of overlapping and interacting triangles within an outer-ringed circle measuring about 80 feet diameter.

Luckily Gill Puttick, who runs the Petersfield Parkinson's help group, gallantly stepped forward to replace Greenwood. Other participants included Essential Tremor sufferer Linda Daubney, former senior reporter of the *Petersfield Herald* and a longtime friend and supporter of my work.

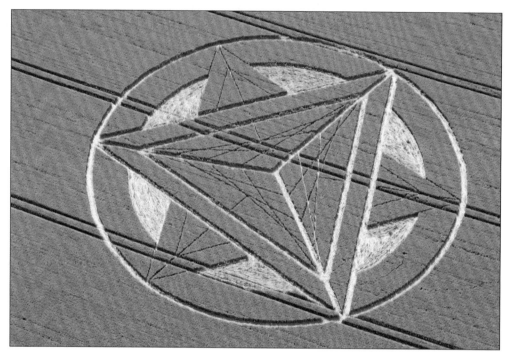

Fig. 8.8. Liddington, Wiltshire, July 1, 2012.

It was a wet day, and we all donned Wellington boots and made our way down the tramlines into the crop circle.

Paul Gerry conducted his tests using a clinical thirty-four-channel EEG machine. As the tests took one hour to set up and record and thirty minutes to remove the glue from the subject's head, only two people were tested, a Parkinson's sufferer and Ann Godden (with restless leg syndrome). Paul Gerry reported:

The equipment records all frequencies up to the "sampling rate," which is set at 256 cycles per second. Then it can digitally filter out any below and above specific values: for example, 0.5–70 Hz is used clinically. I can see the main problem is that an EEG, even when performed on a relaxed subject lying down, still contains a fair amount of muscle artifact, which is high frequency (20-plus Hz).

The technique was as follows: Each subject was recorded from disc electrodes placed according to the 10–20 system, impedances kept below 5 Kohm, glued to the scalp with collodion.

An EEG of fifteen minutes was recorded before in a crop circle and

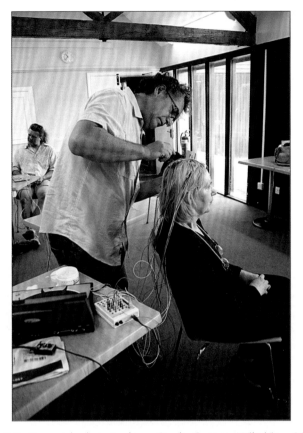

Fig. 8.9. Research day, Avebury Study Centre, Wiltshire, 2012.

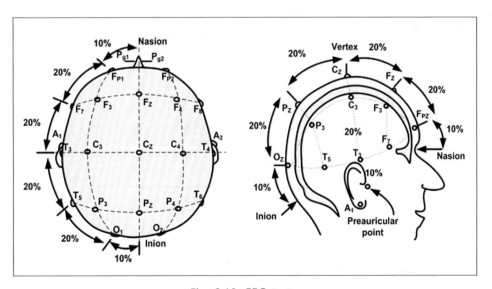

Fig. 8.10. EEG tests.

outside (but within the wheat field) shortly afterward. Each recording included periods of eye opening and eye closure.

After visual inspection an epoch of each of the six recordings was selected (eyes closed, minimal eye movement, and electromyographic artifact).

These samples were analyzed using FFT and frequency maps produced by the psychology department at Leicester University.

As you can see, the result of the procedure (brain mapping) below, over a period of time, is expressed in Power that reads as uV^2 (amplitude squared).

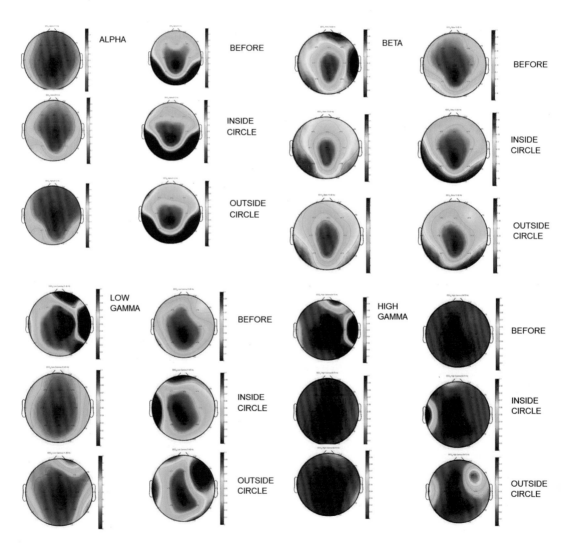

Fig. 8.11. Gamma brain-wave results, before, during, and after visiting the Liddington circle, 2012. Anne's results on the left, Gill's results on the right. Four types of brain waves were measured: alpha, beta, and low and high gamma.

Paul's analysis of Anne's results are shown in figure 8.11 on the left, Gill's on the right, with the following frequencies: alpha 8–12 Hz, beta 13–30 Hz, low gamma 31–45, high gamma 54–70 Hz:

> I leave it to you to make what you will of the results, my comments are that Gill had a good symmetrical alpha rhythm whereas Anne didn't, but little difference occurred suggesting they were in the same states of relaxation. The beta/gamma showing in Anne's "before" over the right mid-temporal area is likely to be slight jaw tension. I can't explain the fast increase in Gill's low and high gamma.

A CONE OF ENERGY

Hazel Drummond reported:

> As soon as we were in the circle I could feel a kind of buzzing and slight heaviness in my legs. I felt a bit uncomfortable as if the energies were slightly negative. I tried using my pendulum and was interested to see that it was turning anticlockwise (negative) no matter where I went in the circle; however, when I went into the center I found that it immediately turned clockwise and did so in a circle around me. Interestingly that was when James Lyons came up and told me that there was a cone of energy rising from that central spot. I felt really well standing in the center. I could have stayed there all day. I felt well and energized—very different from the rest of the circle. After leaving the circle I felt quite woolly-headed, and that continued all day Monday and Tuesday, as often happens after the crop circle day. I also had a horrendously sore throat and no voice on the Sunday evening and Monday but that could have been due to the crop affecting me. By Wednesday I felt back to normal.

With Parkinson's sufferers the brain finds adjusting to narrow spaces a problem, and Gill Puttick had great difficulty walking up the tramline toward the circle. However, after being in the circle, she led the way out of the formation striding along the tramlines without any problems whatsoever. In addition, while inside the circle she had been able to get up out of the floppy canvas-seated chair (not everyone could) but after the double control tests at the perimeter of the field, she was unable to do so.

Puttick reported:

My medication is 2 Symmetrel, each tablet is 100 mg amantadin hydro-chloride. 1 Mirapexin either 2.62 or 2.1—this is prolonged-release prami-pexole. This drug can make you gamble, over-sexed, and many other things. It didn't work for me; it only had a good effect. 1 Madopar 100mg/25mg three times a day. Levodopa + Benserazide.

As for me I've had two good days with lots of energy. Sleep was better even if I did pummel my husband Chris on the shoulder. He was glad his back was toward me; I slept in the other room last night.

Going back to walking through the field. I have a problem with starting off when my meds are low and narrow spaces are a nightmare. It sounds silly but the brain doesn't send the message to the feet to move.

My feet feel very odd; it's like being on ice skates [and] they get quite painful. When the meds switch me on I'm away. I would like to try the circle again with no meds. I would need a driver.

The last two weeks I've had a lot of energy, making birthday cakes for eightieth and ninetieth birthdays. Sorting out a tea party for mother-in-law (ninety), I didn't slow down, walked miles round a steam engine rally in Norfolk.

A BUMPY RIDE

In 2013 we conducted the tests in a lovely crop circle at Overton, part of the famous ancient road called the Ridgeway that stretches from Avebury, Wiltshire, eastward across southern England, passing the Uffington Chalk White Horse on its meandering way before ending up at Beacon Hill in Hertfordshire. The circle consisted of a central circle surrounded by nine rings with a standing center approximately 120 feet in diameter.

Unfortunately clinical physiologist Paul Gerry from the Devon and Exeter Hospital was unable to join us, as a portable EEG was not available. Hazel Drummond of NutriVital Health, who has been a most important longtime part of the team, Parkinson's sufferer Gill Puttick, Dr. Roger Taylor, and myself were the only ones, as James Lyons had mistaken the day and various other mis-haps had befallen the other participants. As it turned out it was just as well, as the trek in 90-degree heat was only for the fittest. Gill Puttick clearly couldn't walk that distance, so I took her in my car. This was a most perilous journey as

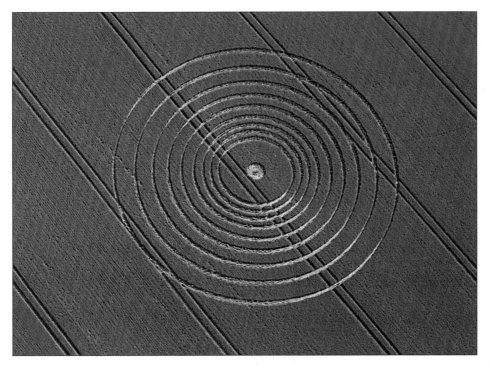

Fig. 8.12. Overton, near Avebury, Wiltshire, July 6, 2013.

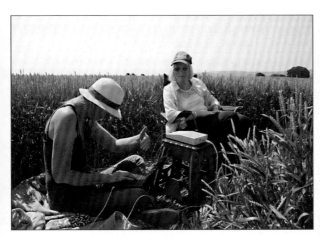

Fig. 8.13. Conducting tests inside and outside the circle at the Overton site, 2013.

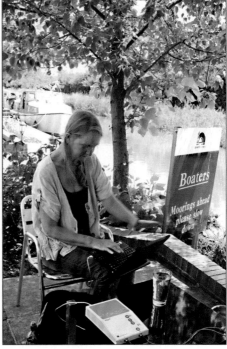

Fig. 8.14. Hazel Drummond at Honey Street in Pewsey Vale, Wiltshire

the track was deeply rutted, ten inches deep in places; getting there we only fell in once, but twice on the way back, and each time I doubted if my car would survive, but survive it did most valiantly. As Gill and I were driving along and still finding no sign of the circle and indeed no chance of seeing it in the flat landscape, we feared that either we had passed it or that we would never find it. Suddenly in a field to our left we saw two people stand up briefly. We had found it, but only because those people had momentarily stood up! Taylor and Drummond joined us on foot, and we walked into the most delightful nine-ringed circle. As I was walking in, I had a sense of music and, knowing that numbers carry frequencies, felt sure that this was what I was "hearing." We conducted the tests in blistering heat. Gill, who had had trouble walking down the tramline, strode out of the field without any problems.

I sent a photograph of the circle to James Lyons and was fascinated by his findings.

> However, this formation is far from simple since it embodies in a remarkable way the key numbers of Earth Energy patterns most certainly including Crop Circles. For some twenty years at least, the number of a circle, namely Pi (3.14159 . . .) is implicit in most formations. A second number Phi (1.6180339 . . .), or the Golden Mean, is also well known, since it is present in all of Nature, including the human form. What is relatively new is the presence of a now well-established constant termed Delta (4.6692 . . .), the first number of Chaos. Since Nature is studied as a dynamic process, it is not surprising to find delta appearing in the Crop Circle scenario. It is the key to understanding the most elusive aspect of the phenomenon—namely, the conscious link.

> [After more discussion he goes on to say,] All these numbers are identifiable within the diatonic music scale. [He ends by saying,] The final point to make is that this formation in such a simple yet elegant form reveals to us the principles of the crop circle phenomenon we have uncovered in the last twenty years or so are fundamentally correct. The Cosmos is all One.

A NEW EXPERIMENT

The year 2014 was another memorable time, and it found us in the most exquisite crop circle of the year, consisting of delicately diminishing spirals that had appeared at Forest Farm only a few minutes north of Marlborough.

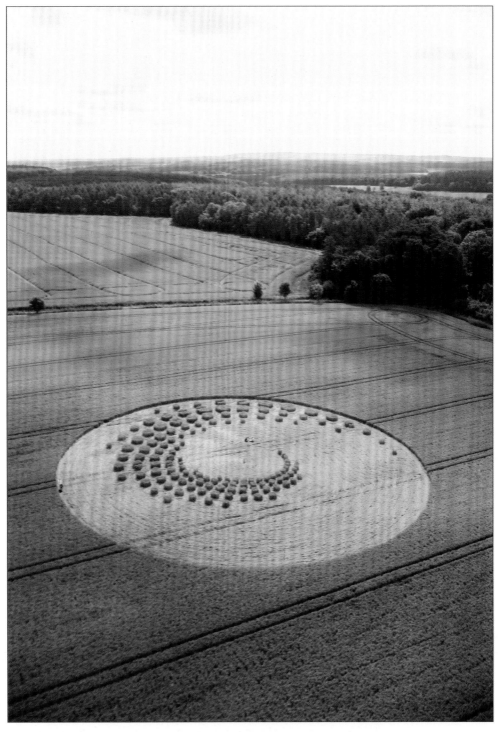

Fig. 8.15. Forest Farm, near Marlborough, Wiltshire,
July 16, 2014.

Gill Puttick was with us once again when we visited this circle, as was Tina Martin, an Essential Tremor sufferer.

This was an experimental day as the circle had been harvested two days before we conducted our tests, but I was of the opinion that the "energy" would still be present in the fallen crop and indeed this proved to be the case, as the results showed.

As always we started the day by conducting tests at the Avebury Study Centre.

The Parkinson's tests this year were ones recommended by a neurologist and especially aimed at this condition. They were carried out by Paul Gerry, who was once again with us. Our guinea pigs were Gill Puttick, who had been with me for three years; Tim Challoner, who refuses to take any medication; and Tina Martin. In addition Paul tested several other non-sufferers, including Angie Kibble, James Lyons, and me.

Among the tests were

1. Glabella tap test. This is a primitive reflex where the eyes shut if an individual is tapped lightly between the eyebrows. This reflex may normally be overcome rapidly—that is, the individual soon fails to blink—usually in less than five taps. In a patient with frontal release signs the reflex cannot be overcome, and they continue to blink for as long as the examiner cares to keep tapping. A similar response is seen with late Parkinsonism.

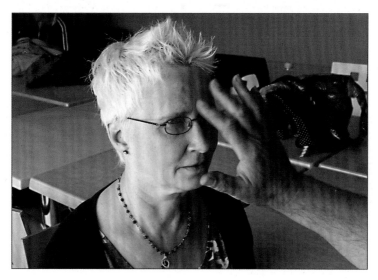

Fig. 8.16. Administering the Glabella tap test
at scientific research day, 2014.

2. Timed dot and cross test. This entails using a tablet computer in which the program is installed, and where the person being tested moves their finger as fast and accurately as they can from one dot to the other in a timed period.

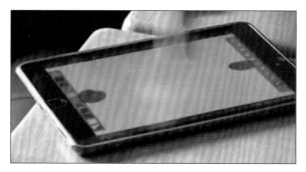

Fig. 8.17. The timed dot and cross test.

3. A vibration sensor designed by the Parkinsonism trust that gives a frequency distribution graph and peak frequency when holding a mobile phone for a given length of time.

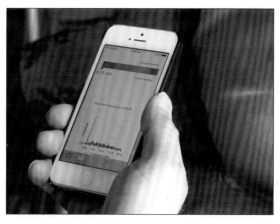

Fig. 8.18. A vibration sensor for Parkinson's disease patients.

Tim Challoner wrote after visiting the circle at Forest Farm:

I was diagnosed with Parkinson's just over one year ago. I have been to the doctor and specialist about the condition, but I have chosen not to go on medication. Instead I take natural, mostly Neways, products.

My condition expresses itself in the form of lack of energy, a little shaking (tremors), and difficulty in sleeping. Also part of my condition expresses itself in lack of facial expression and a little difficulty in enunciating words.

My body can be rigid at times and moving can be labored. Despite this I believe my thinking is sharp, and I remain positive and open to any help with my condition.

Yesterday within the circle, I felt relaxed and at peace, on the way home I was sleepy. I think it is too early to say if there has been a shift for the better. But I do hope there is a circle that has an energy that will make a difference.

MY HAND STOPPED SHAKING

Tina Martin wrote:

As a bit of background, I have a Familial Essential Tremor. This has been in three generations of my family (and maybe more but I do not have that information). My tremor was at a very low level up to six years ago when, in a period of stress, it worsened. I am a painter, and teach painting, and since this worsening I now do all my art work with my left (nondominant) hand and most tasks also. The tremor is in my dominant right hand chiefly, and at a low, occasional, level in my head. I take a very low dose of a beta-blocker for this, Propranolol, 20 mg a day. I am unable to increase this dose, as it affects my blood pressure.

The major thing I noticed in the circle was that my right hand (which had been shaking very badly when the initial tests were done) was completely still. Looking at the two hands there was no difference between them. The right hand is never completely still like that, and I commented on it at the time. Thinking about it now, I think I would have liked to do a writing test before, within, and out of the circle. It would have been interesting to see if the effect showed in the writing, and maybe how long the effect lasted.

This handwriting test suggested by Tina is an excellent one, easy to do, and easy to interpret. (See pages 151 and 152 for more details.)

WHAT HAPPENED TO THE WATER?

Gill Puttick recounted:

I was still on the same medication at this time. My day started with a phone call at 7:20 from Lucy just checking if I'm awake. I'd been up since 6:10 a.m.

I arrived at Lucy's just before 8:00. A good start to an informative day out.

Hazel set up and did her test. She said my ears and tubes were not happy; I awoke next day with a sore throat. The test also showed I was unbalanced.

Paul Gerry tapped my forehead, had me tapping his tablet and holding his mobile phone.

I had a chat with Tim, who also has Parkinson's but not on any medication; I would have liked a longer chat. Tim has made up his mind he doesn't want medication; that's his choice but he could feel so much better and have a quality of life.

We set off for the circle. I will admit to being a bit of a skeptic, but this time I saw dowsing rods move in the same place every time. Whilst watching this I took a sip of my water; it was warm. I walked across the circle and took another sip expecting it to be warm only to find it was cold. Now explain that one to me.

Hazel did her test again in the circle only to find I was balanced again; this surprised us both. Paul did his test.

ENCOURAGING RESULTS

Paul Gerry's results were one of the most illustrative of any we have had in the past. They showed clearly the differences between the Parkinson's and Essential Tremor volunteers and the non-sufferers.

In particular after the first control tests at Avebury Study Centre and subsequently both inside the circle and later outside the circle (second control tests), the reduction of tremor by 18 percent and 15 percent during the second control tests is a dramatic revelation (fig. 8.19). This is most exciting, and shows us that we can in the future use freshly cut-out crop circles for our tests.

Also conducting scientific tests in 2014 was Hazel Drummond of NutriVital Health, who has generously given her time and energy to this research for many years using the renowned Asyra (Quest 4) technique, which covers a broad spectrum of investigation and consists of various tests as listed below.

1. **Baseline test:** this test measures energy states in major organs and systems. This can give an indication of which organs are out of balance and could indicate health problems.
2. **Comprehensive test:** thousands of test items in the computer's database are tested to show whether one has been affected by viruses,

PERCENTAGE CHANGES FROM INITIAL CONTROL DATA		
IN CIRCLE	**CONTROL GROUP**	**SUBJECT AVERAGE**
Tap	10% better	5% better
Tremor	2.7% lower	18% lower
Touch	15% better	11% better
EDGE OF FIELD		
Tap	43% better	10% better
Tremor	2.3% lower	15% lower
Touch	21% better	12% better

Fig. 8.19. Control test results from Paul Gerry
for inside and outside the crop circle.

bacteria, parasites, and so forth. We run three tests: the initial tests in the Avebury Study Centre, next identical tests inside the circle, and the third identical one outside the circle. These three identical tests are compared and analyzed.

3. **Hormonal imbalance in the endocrine system:** Thirty-one hormonal signatures are tested for imbalances.
4. **Neurotransmitters.**
5. **Brain-wave patterns.**
6. **Vertebral misalignments.**
7. **Meridian disturbances.**
8. **Electrolyte disturbances.**
9. **Chakra imbalances:** the seven chakras are tested.
10. **Geopathic stress and harmful energies:** This part of the testing protocol looks at one's exposure to Earth Energy fields, electromagnetic stress, mineral deposits, power lines, microwave energies, radioactive exposure, ultraviolet waves, and X-rays.

Drummond's results mirrored Gerry's results. There were four people showing quite severe imbalances initially in the Avebury Study Centre control tests—the three Parkinson's and Essential Tremor sufferers and me. The fact that I showed up so detrimentally illustrated the stress and tension I had been under! However, inside the circle our results showed quite marked improvement.

On the other hand, whereas Emily Weeks felt great before entering the formation, she was the only person to feel really ill inside the circle, and this

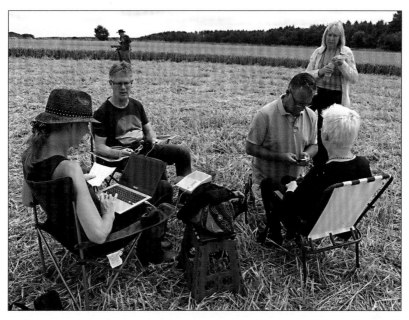

Fig. 8.20. Scientific research day, Forest Farm,
near Marlborough, Wiltshire, 2014.

was clearly demonstrated by Drummond's results by showing up as imbalance in the baseline tests.

This turned out to be a pioneering experimental day and one that reaped more unusual results than on many previous occasions. One of the most interesting things about the circle was that none of the participants seemed to notice that the standing pattern had been cut out, perhaps because so many strange effects were being felt and monitored.

I WAS THROWN OFF THE SPOT

While inside the circle I experienced an effect never felt before. Clairvoyant Mona da Silva came up to me and told me that she had found a certain spot in the circle on which she could not keep her balance and kept being thrown off. Fascinated, I followed her and after a bit she found the exact spot (no mean achievement in a 200-foot-diameter circle). Was it really happening? I stepped onto it and was immediately rocked backward a couple of steps. I tried it several times with exactly the same result. What was happening? Was it due to some vortical energy? Maybe we will never know. If anyone has also experienced this effect, please write to let me know.

Mona described her experience in the circle thus:

I felt at the spot I showed you—it was as if I was in water at the beach where you stand and are rocked back and forth and lose balance where you feel rising and swaying down again. This became more intense after about a minute—I was in a "meditative" mode. I could see colors in my head—intense violet cerise to red—it felt warm to be in. It felt as if I was within a living organism. I know that in the bright sunshine I saw Paul Craddock's body almost as a silhouette—that was the bright Sun/glare with the clear shape of his hat—but with this figure this was not the case, it was different.

I shut my eyes and just followed the "flow." I have to say that when I was at the watery feel end I did turn to the left and felt there was energy drawing on the other end in a line, or should I say, a large block/oblong range. However, walking as I did, which was with eyes shut and feeling my way somewhat random/circular, I ended in the second spot where the energy was so much stronger—intense red and orange-pink colors in my head—staying longer it altered to being golden and then pearlescent/rainbow flecks. It was this spot I

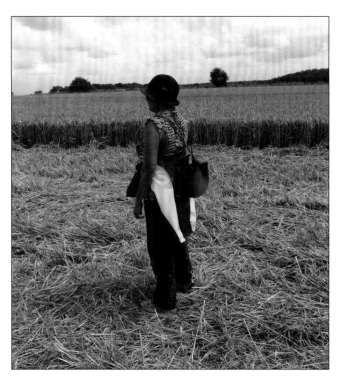

Fig. 8.21. Mona standing in the center of the circle,
Forest Farm, near Marlborough, Wiltshire, 2014.

pointed out to Paul, Tim, and so on. It seemed to be a small circular shape on the ground but that was not my awareness when going there—we only noticed later. Also, that position was in an alignment with the previous spot on the right, and not a spot but a position that kept shifting slightly for both "spots." Though I felt it was like a long chunk of energy flow within that alignment.

I can still connect with that amazing energy, and I thank you for letting us share this with you and all the wonderful people there—not least all who tested Tim—I know he felt the benefit of the experience too.

The other thing I noticed was how restful and calm it felt in the circle; time seemed to stand still and it was a very relaxing feel.

Asyra (Quest 4) expert Hazel Drummond reported that "I felt very happy in the circle . . . very calm and balanced. I felt happy and would have loved to have stayed longer. Stephen actually admitted to me that he felt a bit nauseous and a bit headachy in the circle, which really surprised him, as he didn't expect to feel anything. This passed off after leaving the circle though."

MY FIRST EXPERIENCE

And finally, Angie Kibble, who was tested by Gerry alongside James Lyons and me, told me:

It was my first experience of being in a crop circle; I didn't know quite what to expect despite having read several books on the subject over the years. When I am out dowsing on Dartmoor quite often I am able to pick up energy lines without using dowsing rods as I experience a kind of buzzing sensation in my head—for want of a better description—when I cross them. When I reached the center of the crop circle on Sunday I was aware of a similar sensation, which seemed stronger in certain areas, to the extent that I became quite nauseous and felt the need to move away from what seemed to be the source of the sensation. I lay down on the edge of the crop circle for some minutes, which felt a bit better, and whilst looking up at the sky I was aware of lots of tiny dancing pinpricks of light, which appeared to be multicolored. This was very different to the odd "floating" specks you occasionally see going across your eyes when drifting off to sleep, and was rather lovely.

When you walked me around the crop circle to a different spot I did feel a little better, but it wasn't until we left the circle and walked right away that

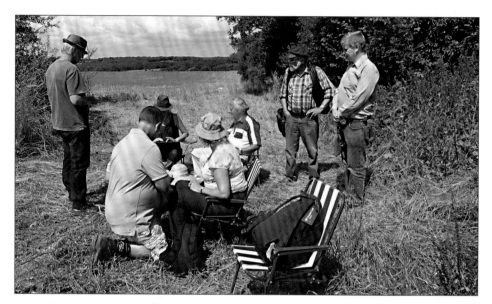

Fig. 8.22. Conducting control test outside the circle, Forest Farm, near Marlborough, Wiltshire, 2014.

I felt completely all right again. I noticed that I felt very energized for several hours afterward, but by the evening I was so weary I didn't know where to put myself. Being a novice I am not sure if this is a standard reaction!

So as not to influence the test results until all the tests had been conducted, participants are encouraged to drink only water to avoid dehydration. As we had not eaten since breakfast time our tummies were rumbling, but at last we repaired, as the previous year, to the charming Honey Street Café, run and owned by a dedicated and hardworking young couple, Joe and Sophie. Lying alongside the canal and close to and beneath the Alton Barnes Chalk White Horse, it is a perfect place to relax in their wonderfully comfortable wicker armchairs and enjoy not only the delicious home-cooked food but the perfectly landscaped summer garden. Here we discussed our preliminary results and experiences before going our separate ways.

Gill Puttick reported: "I struggled walking into the circle, but managed to walk out leading the way."

Essential Tremor sufferer Tina Martin wrote:

The major thing I noticed in the circle was that my right hand (which had been shaking very badly when the initial tests were done) was completely still. My right hand is never completely still like that. I would have liked to do a writing test before, within, and out of the circle to see if the effect showed in the writing, and maybe how long the effect lasted.

A SYMBOL OF LOVE

Her wish was granted when in 2015 we conducted our tests (see page 152), using the same program as before, when we visited the circle that turned out to be one of my favorites of all time, the beautiful Uffcott "Rose" near Wroughton in Wiltshire. Appearing on midsummer's day, it was a joy to behold.

As always, we carried out the same research procedure by conducting preliminary tests at Avebury Study Centre, then tests inside the circle, and later a second control test some distance from the circle.

The story behind this circle is a poignant one. In November 2014 the farmer James Hussey, who owns this field and the surrounding land, lost his lovely wife, Gill, after a fourteen-year battle with breast cancer. I knew her well, and she was a most lovely lady with a huge love and respect for the circles. They had always generously allowed people to visit the circles on their land. They were a most devoted couple.

The field where this circle appeared was one where Gill used to ride regularly, and somehow it seemed fitting that this glorious crop circle depicting a rose should find its resting place just there. As we all know, the rose is a symbol of love, among other things, so what clearer message could Gill have sent her

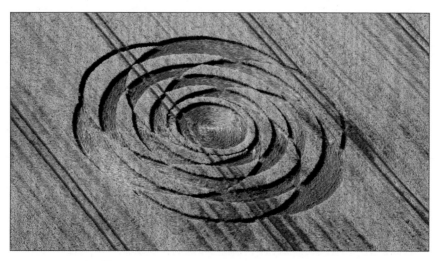

Fig. 8.23. Uffcott Rose, near Wroughton, Wiltshire, June 22, 2015.

husband James? Even if I didn't know that the rose is a symbol of love, the strength of love emanating from the frequencies that radiate and pour out of this photograph are overwhelming.

To the ancient Egyptians the rose was sacred to Isis, and the ancient Greeks and Romans identified the rose with the goddess of love, Aphrodite (Greek name) or Venus (Roman name).

Islam and Sufism also considered the rose to be a symbol of love, using it in geometric gardens where it held pride of place. The rose's association with the song of the nightingale was considered to have been inspired by love and by the beauty of the rose, as portrayed in the poems of Hafez.

Medieval Christians identified the five petals of the rose with the five wounds of Christ, and a red rose as a symbol of love—often given to a loved one on Valentine's Day.

We frequently see wonderful rose windows in churches and cathedrals comprising five or ten segments (the five petals and five sepals of a rose). The rose is the national flower of England, and Henry VII used it to create the Tudor rose, which combined the red and white roses of the noble Houses of Lancaster and York.

Indeed, the rose universally depicts Love, so what greater tribute could Gill Hussey have sent not just to James but also to everyone? James set up a charity to raise money for a breast-screening unit in Swindon as the closest unit was in Oxford, and for Gill and others to have to travel many hours for a daily treatment lasting a few minutes each time over a period of six weeks was altogether too exhausting and draining. Everyone who visited the rose and later the "Thunder Bird" crop circle gave generously to the fund, and James, by

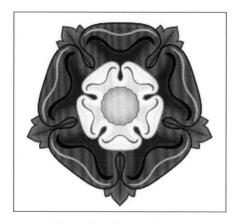

Fig. 8.24. The Tudor Rose.

organizing events such as marathons, was able to raise almost £10,000. This was a fitting testimony to Gill's love of life, James, and people in general. (For more information visit www.justgiving.com/Gill-Hussey.)

THE MIND MIRROR SYSTEM

With James's permission, this was the circle we used for our 2015 scientific research day. He kindly left it unharvested so that we could conduct the tests. As usual we began the day at Avebury Study Centre, which is well equipped with plenty of power outlets. Paul Gerry, clinical physiologist from Devon and Exeter Hospital, kindly joined us once again, and NutriVital Health expert Hazel Drummond was also there to conduct the scientific tests. Gerry was using the new MM (Multi-Mirror) system, which is a highly complex machine that, in addition to testing for brain activity, can record a person's autonomic system (this is measuring parts of our body that are not under our control, such as heartbeat, intestines, movements of the pupil of the eye, and chemistry of the blood).

In figure 8.26 (page 144), on the far right of the screen are traffic lights giving indication of quality of signal; green means strong. To the left of the lights is the Mind Mirror shape, with the highest frequency at the top. On the top left are the raw brain-wave traces. Bottom left is a frequency spectrum, which gives frequency (vertical axis) and time (horizontal axis), and color is the amount—yellow is large amount. Gerry was measuring what was happening to their brains over five-minute periods while resting their heads against

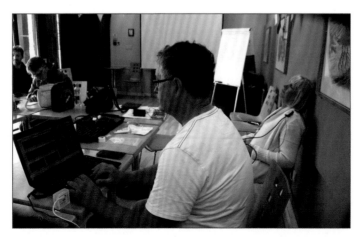

Fig. 8.25. Crop-circle research day, Avebury Study Centre, Wiltshire, 2015.

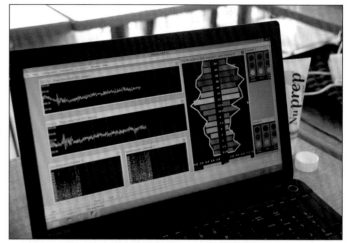

Fig. 8.26. The Mind Mirror used by Paul Gerry.

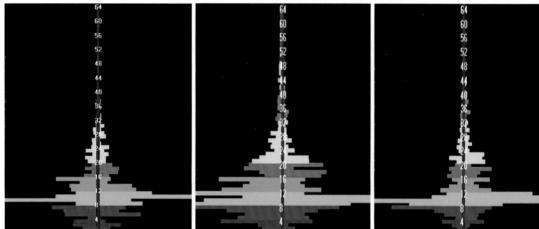

Fig. 8.27. (a) Gamma levels before entering the crop circle, (b) gamma levels inside the crop circle, (c) gamma levels after leaving the crop circle.

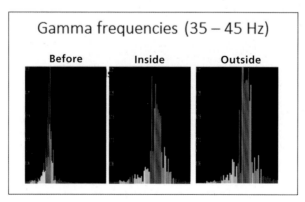

Fig. 8.28. Gamma frequencies before, inside, and after leaving the crop circle.

the wall with eyes closed. Gerry tested James and Gill Puttick, Tina Martin, and Mona da Silva. Figures 8.27 and 8.28 show the three changes for Mona before our excursion to the circle, inside the circle, and then outside the circle, respectively. The orange depicts the gamma levels. The analysis of these tests is complete.

As she had on previous research days, Hazel Drummond used the Asyra technique and generously gave her time and energy to this research. The Asyra technique covers a broad spectrum of investigation, and it is fascinating to look back and see how the technology and methodology has improved. Parkinson's disease sufferers Gill Puttick and Tim Challoner (accompanied by clairvoyant Mona) together with Essential Tremor sufferer Tina Martin all gallantly put themselves forward to be tested again. Gill also brought along her son James who is suffering from an as-yet-undiagnosed condition of extreme fatigue syndrome, which has steadily grown worse over the last few years. Also with us was Hazel's husband, Stephen. They had driven all the way from Manchester, setting off at the crack of sparrows that morning.

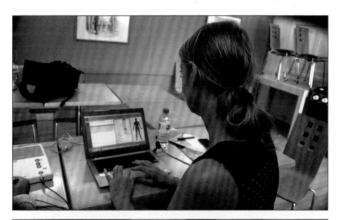

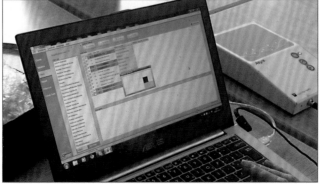

Fig. 8.29. Asyra testing done on scientific research day, 2015.

We then proceeded to the rose formation at Uffcott conveniently close to Avebury. As the circle was already three weeks old, I was concerned that it would be past its best.

Despite the dire warnings of wet weather, the day turned out to be roasting hot with not a drop of rain. As we drove down the narrow road to Uffcott I was not altogether sure in which field the crop circle lay, so as we neared the area, as far as I could remember seeing it from the air, I asked James Puttick, who is over six feet tall, to get out and stand on a hay bale at a gap in the hedge. This is what he wrote:

> As we left the center and traveled toward the circle I was suffering the disorientation I always feel when traveling by car through country that is new to me. After ten minutes of driving and navigating we arrived in the general area of the circle, but we did not know its actual location. I jumped out of the car, and as soon as my feet touched the ground my disorientation was instantly gone! I instantly knew my location and could feel where the circle was—it was like a low frequency buzz through the ground—I could feel it. I turned toward it and looked through a gap in the hedge, I could not see it, so I jumped on a bale and looked where I knew it was and still couldn't see it.
>
> I was sort of miffed I couldn't see it because I knew at a base level that was where it was in the field. So I looked along the hedge line from where I was and saw a person a little further along next to a vehicle. I knew we were meeting the farmer (who kindly allowed the circle to remain) at this location, so I returned to the car and we parked up. This is where my day got strange.

We made our way into the field and, on reaching the circle, we dowsed for the area of strongest "energy." It became clear that in the lower part of the circle closest to the road, there were a series of strong vortices rendering several of us quite dizzy and unsteady. Both Paul and Hazel set up their instruments and the tests were repeated. We stayed in the circle for some time making further investigations. It was clear that this was a formation containing unusually high "energies," and I was relieved that I had not taken our group in when it was fresher, as I believe the "energies" would have been too great, especially for those of us who are "sensitive." We met James Hussey at the edge of the field on leaving. He was interested to hear how we had got on and what had happened.

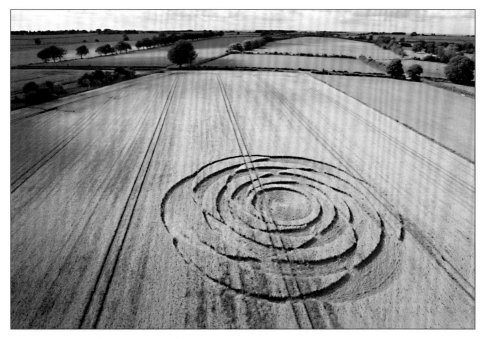

Fig. 8.30. Uffcott Rose, near Wroughton, Wiltshire, June 22, 2015.

We conducted the second control tests further down the road near the hedge. Unusually, Hazel's battery had been completely drained by the circle, so she made her way to the local pub where she was allowed to plug into their electrical system and finish the tests. We all met up there, and it was clear to us that this had been no ordinary circle. Here are some of the other interesting reports I was sent.

Hazel reported:

Because the crop circle that we were about to visit was over three weeks old I had no expectations of any "energetic" disturbances affecting me. Over the years of going with Lucy on the research days, some circles have had very strong energies, which have sometimes made me feel ill for a few days after. Some have not affected me at all.

I was about halfway from the entrance to the field and the circle when it suddenly hit me. I felt a very strong weakness and trembly feeling through-out my whole body. The feeling took me by surprise, and it grew stron-ger as we reached the inside of the circle. I felt a sort of whirling energy that was incredibly strong. I didn't particularly want to sit down in it but thought that it would be good to do the testing at such a strong energetic point and will be interested to see the results on all of the test subjects. I continued with that strong trembly feeling until we left the circle and didn't feel any particular aftereffects except that I felt very well that week.

At one point during the afternoon I walked around the circle with rods and was again struck by the force of the energy and noted that there were definite points around the circle where it was even stronger and where the arms of the rods were twisting through 360 degrees and even spinning around again.

James Puttick's story continued:

The day had started with a jump when I was woken early with yells of "We're going earlier, get a move on!" This is not the way of a normal Sunday. On arriving at the Avebury Study Centre I was a bit more awake than in the first hours of the day, I found the science used fascinating. It was great to talk with everyone in a more relaxed setting, and to learn more about the circles and the land where they occur. I was aware of both Paul and Hazel's methods, and I understood the principles behind them, but this was the first time that I had seen them being used in front of me. The results of my tests on Hazel's equipment were very surprising and highlighted one problem in my body that I had suspected for a while but my doctor had told me to ignore.

I felt energized as I entered the circle, my mind cleared, my body felt light and supple, for the first time all day I felt great, none of the usual body aches and tiredness. This continued for about thirty minutes after we left the circle, but then I crashed as we were doing the last tests at the interim stop, my body felt heavy again but my mind was still clearer than at the start of the day.

After I had sat down for a few minutes at the river my mind started to get foggy again, and I noticed I was getting confused whilst talking to people. It was only then that I realized that all the time I was in the circle and the time just after leaving it, how good I felt and how clear my mind was. I cannot explain this effect.

It is interesting to note that many "sensitive" people find that the circles increase this effect. Mona da Silva wrote telling me this interesting series of subsequent events:

I had an extreme reaction for about five days afterward—my eyes were very sore and constantly watering—I was told that this was due to hay fever by the doctor. It started when I was in the crop circle and I just kept wiping my eyes—did not think about it. The last time I went the crop had been harvested (2014 crop circle tests). However, I have been near hay before and not had such an extreme reaction.

Whilst there I was aware of the energy from the mast, however, when walking to the circle and on entering the periphery there was a strong draw toward the crop circle. The energy felt different to the crop circle last year—with this one there was the moving up and down of energy almost like being on soft waves of the sea when swimming, under one's feet and yet the areas where it happened also seem to be moving in swirls.

I know that there were tests taken before and after, one of which was the writing in the circle, and I certainly could not write properly on the paper. Also the measurements taken from your colleague (Paul or Hazel?). I know that at the end test we aborted the results as the measurement was not so easy to conduct. I do think that it may also have been me—I do meditate and can go into higher frequency—my definition of going into theta as a practicing ThetaHealer I think might be different from what is being measured.

When we finished at the pub with final measurements and drinks, etc., I then got into the car to drive off. I think you came over to check when you found I had stopped further down the road—at a time when I was checking the GPS, which did not appear to be operating properly. As we were parked, the others drove off too, overtaking us, and finally we were able to pull out and drive off too. I had to turn off some 200 yards and it was soon after that I can only describe seeing opaque/white forms, about the height of a child maybe 2 to 3 feet and it was the sound of them speaking that I remember—a language I could not make out—I was driving and had to tune out. It was like they flashed in front of me talking to each other and directing to me and flashed out again, about three or four, I think.

Now please do not think me weird or unhinged. Last week I did some further work with Theta and linking to minerals, crystals, and plants. It was not until I was about to fall asleep that it suddenly clicked that when I tuned in to the plant, which was a growing orchid, I heard a language and realized that it was similar to what I had heard from the opaque forms. Their heads were larger than ours and rounder and maybe a third in length to their body—two arms and two legs—reminding me of the form of paper cutout figures.

The figure I saw last year was different; the energy from the form was more authoritative or assured, heading toward me with purpose and I tuned out. I described it as having a long body and very tall and having a very large head shaped like an old-fashioned keyhole.

After having visited the crop circle last year, very soon after I experienced at odd times in the night flashing lights by the kitchen window and even by a very large window on the landing, and Tim felt it by one of the bedrooms—the energy was quite overwhelming and actually quite scary—I really felt vulnerable. This was not passing car lights; it was higher in the sky. At about this time I came across Andara crystals and found them to have energy that helped and what I felt was more divine and full of light; this seemed to help dissipate what I had been encountering.

This time, with this crop circle and what I experienced with the child-like forms, the energy was very different like curious playful chattering, not overwhelming. What I can say is that I have noted a connection with "crop circle" and "plant" in the language I tuned in too. Please note I had not tried to tune in to any plant before, it was part of training I was doing with Theta only last week. Tim has said that he could not stay in the center; the energy was so strong it was making him feel sick. I will type anything else he may want to add tomorrow—send it very quickly to you.

I admire you for how you continue to keep up the good work! If ever you go up again in a helicopter to see a crop circle, please ask me, I would be interested—only ever had one flying lesson—would love to be able to fly a plane on my own. Now would that not be fun?

Tim sensed there were a number of vortices around the circular walkway, that is, the flattened crop. He felt relaxed in the center of the circle but not on the periphery where the flattened walkway was going to the outside of the circle. Jennifer Percival, who runs a training course for the NHS, wrote:

Thank you for asking me to attend this year's research event. It was a very interesting day!

In terms of aftereffects from visiting the circle—I wanted to let you know that I became very tired and felt exhausted as the afternoon wore on. This is highly unusual for me. I also slept for ten hours that night, which I haven't done in years, so I guess this was to do with my time in the circle's energy field.

On closer analysis, Hazel Drummond's results revealed an interesting pattern. "Seven of the nine showed a noticeably increased imbalance inside the circle as compared to first control tests at the Avebury Study Centre. This imbalance was maintained in four of the nine in the second control tests outside the circle."

In addition, five of the nine showed a change in hypothalamus levels. The hypothalamus is a very important part of the forebrain, which lies below the thalamus and forms the lower part of the ventricle and its floor. Its integrity is essential to life. As noted above, it plays a major part in regulation of the temperature of the body, body weight, and appetite, sexual behavior and rhythms, blood pressure, and fluid balance, and it is suggested that it could even be said to be the physical basis of the emotions.

In figure 8.31, the blue lines are the first tests conducted at the Avebury Study Centre, the orange lines show repeat tests taken inside the circle, and the gray lines are double-control tests conducted outside the circle. Taking 60 as the norm, you can see how the orange lines fluctuated.

The change in Tina's writing was quite dramatic, especially as she did not have anything hard on which to press when writing inside the circle. However, as you can see in figure 8.32 (page 152), the deterioration over the following days was noticeable. Tina mentioned that she found trying to draw a spiral was one of the most difficult things she attempted. Straight lines were also a problem.

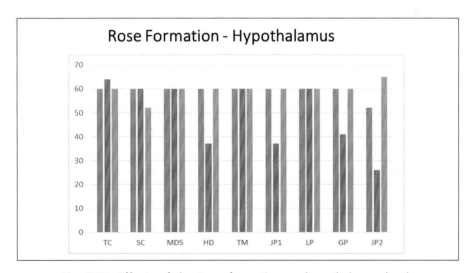

Fig. 8.31. Effects of the Rose formation on hypothalamus levels of the nine participants.

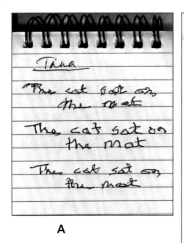

A

B

C

Fig. 8.32. Effects of the crop circles on Tina's handwriting: (a) before going into the crop circle, (b) inside the crop circle, (c) after leaving the crop circle.

A PLASMA WALL

On July 23, three Spanish tourists visited the formation not knowing that it had already been harvested. On reaching the edge of field they realized that they were unable to see where the circle had been. According to researcher Charles Mallett, "The three stood there looking into the field for remnants of the circle when suddenly they noticed a 'tornado' of spinning crop and dirt down the field about 115 meters [350 feet] from where they were standing."

They could see dirt and dust debris from the field appearing more or less in the middle of the field. They described a very large, spinning tornado focused at the center of the crop circle and then going up 60 to 70 feet. They went into the field straight to where the tornado was happening, and as they approached it seemed that the tornado was coming up from the flattened ground and they then found themselves in the clearly defined flattened site where the circle had been. The flattened crop was still lying unharvested. The tornado seemed to be emanating from the exact center where the crop circle had been. After a short time the tornado moved away and disappeared. At that point two of them decided to return to their car, leaving just one Spaniard inside the circle.

The remaining tourist then noticed another "tornado" forming on the ground at her feet—starting very small—then rising up in front of her about two feet away. And as she stood there, this tiny spinning vortex of air and dirt and dust lifted up out of the ground in front of her and rose up what she said was about 11 to 12 meters (36 to 40 feet) in height; this rapidly spinning column of air was very hot.

She said the air started to move from her right to her left around her slightly and never actually enveloped her. This vortex-like effect of "hot" spinning air and dirt then started to move around the circle then away from it at some speed, then more or less curled off and started to drift away down the field—at which point the witness decided to follow it . . . and she described it accelerating, starting slowly and then moving quite rapidly, and it was drifting off toward a field of maize-like sweet corn. She tried to follow it. She started to run as this thing was picking up speed, a twelve-meters-high [39 feet] vortex of spinning air and dirt rushing off down the field. As she moved toward the effect she saw immediately in front of her an almost invisible, almost transparent, but not quite a wall of what she described as energy, a pressure wave, almost transparent but it physically stopped her in her tracks when she was trying to follow this tornado.

That wall stayed rigidly in place for some moments and then the tornado disappeared down the field and cut into the maize field and this wall of energy had a watery, glassy wall effect—you know when you blow children's soap bubbles, they have this glossy, shimmering kind of colored effect?

She was absolutely clear that she could see and pretty much feel, in a sense, this barrier that seemed to be stopping her. And all of this emanating from pretty much the center of a harvested crop circle. Once the tornado had disappeared, the wall disappeared.

This report reminded me of the time that Ray Barnes, who lives at Westbury, Wiltshire (and who was one of the first people to ever witness a crop circle form), described another strange event. On the evening of Thursday, July 26, 1990, he was walking toward the field in which he had seen a circle appear several years before, when he noticed that

there was a heath fire somewhere toward the west and the smoke from it was blowing across the field. The smoke was so dense that I couldn't see the sky through it. But then something caught my attention. Halfway across the field it was as if a glass "wall" had been erected. The smoke blew and billowed against the wall, but apparently could not cross it. To the left of the barrier the air was clear, and the sky and clouds could be seen.

What possible explanation could there be for these two similar events? I consulted James Lyons who, when I read out the description of the tornado "wall," said he had never heard such a brilliant layman's description of the following. He explained that

matter occurs in four phases—Gas, Liquid, Solid, and Plasma. Of these by far the most abundant is Plasma, which occupies 99.9 percent of the Cosmos. This form is seen most often in kitchen lighting or neon signs. It occurs naturally in Nature being the "shells" that cover ancient sites and crop circles. They appear like soap bubbles sitting on a flat surface. Their structure was discovered in 1927 by Langmuir who named these electric shells "Double Layers." Plasma consists of positive and negative charge, similar to the terminals of a battery. The electric field can be extremely strong. Vortex centers in the Earth, which give rise to tornado-like spinning electric charges, generate these hemispherical shells of such large radius (hundreds of meters) that they appear to be wall-like. They can be cloudy or shimmer like soap bubbles. People sense these at ancient sites and elsewhere where strong vortex centers occur. They are in effect akin to the human Aura that many people can "see" and/or "feel."

Such shells are often seen associated with tornadoes. If the vorticity is so great then people sense them as almost solid walls.

The research will continue on an annual basis, and if this work can in any way make a solid contribution to the furtherance of our understanding and curing of Parkinson's disease that would be a tribute to everyone involved and to the crop circles themselves. I hope that in time we may get sponsoring.

COMMENTS BY JAMES LYONS

We have touched on many of the factors that influence the crop-circle creation process and, indeed, the resulting health effects on all animals, including ourselves. Yet it is not just the crop circle phenomenon that is under critical scrutiny; the very foundations of current science from the cosmic to the quantum worlds is in dire straits. From the Big Bang via Dark Matter to Black Holes—all is being rigorously reassessed. Black Holes are now no longer claimed to be dramatic cosmic sinkholes, they are now termed "Gray." Why? Because it has been at last detected that columnar vortices emerge from their polar regions.

These holes are located at the center of Galaxies of which there are literally uncountable numbers. These Galaxies have usually four arms that emerge from the Galactic center as spiraling cones made of individual stars.

Not in the least surprising is that this basic structural layout is modeled in the crop circle world by the well-known Stonehenge formation, the Julia Set, observed by many bystanders forming over a time period of around twenty-five minutes. There are some 150 individual circles involved. This overall pattern is synonymous with the generic structure of a Galaxy. Additionally, the hemispherical cloud over the formation with a clear gap between its lower surface and the ground mimics precisely the form we see in the creation process of many Galaxies. It is so true to say: As above, so below. This formation process has everything to do with the creation of all matter, including ourselves.

Let us remind ourselves that there are only two topological structures that are relevant to all creation: the torus (think of a finger ring) and a spherical shell (like a Ping-Pong ball). Around these are wound spirals of filamentary structures. They can be cross-wound such that we have right-hand and left-hand spirals, often interleaved. All told they form a toroid.

The whole result looks just like a ball of string with its central hole.

It is not in the least surprising to find that this form is key to Yogic Science and is indeed the universal physical atom discovered by Leadbeater and Besant over a century ago. It is the form of everyone's auric field. Not surprisingly, all atomic particles can be modeled in this way as waves around toroids.

We find this form in stone circles. The classic example is Castlerigg, whose ground pattern follows precisely the geometry of a single wave wrapped around a toroidal energy form whose center hole is the thickness of the ring. We find these forms in volcanoes and dolphin rings as well as fairy rings.

It is the interleaving of the right- and left-hand spirals that dictates the effect of Earth Energies on living things. Males and females are created by the spiraling energy fields in their right- and left-brain hemispheres. It is the frequency modulation of these two nested waves that determines the state of health of individuals. The basic nesting of these spirals, like one Slinky inside a larger outer one, dictates all living matter. It is the basic structure of the Birkeland currents that pervade the Cosmos.

We thus arrive at the key point with regard to health effects in crop circles. The whole crop circle is created within a hemispherical shell. There are columnar vortices made up of nested spiraling columns of energy not unlike tornados. These spiraling energies are modulated with frequencies that are resonant with Earth Energies such as 28 kHz, but there is a spectrum of sub-frequencies down to the Schumann resonance of around 8 Hz. It is the spectrum of frequencies that exists in crop circles that interact with the human body and brain. As this book is being written, it is only just becoming possible to analyze the spectrum of these frequencies within the brain. This process is absolutely essential to the understanding of how these specific frequencies interact with humans in particular.

The latest Mind Mirror equipment has the ability to undertake a complete analysis of brain frequencies involved. This should enable us, even in the near future, to start to comprehend how the energy interacts with the body. We expect from now on to be able to compile graphical material that indicates what frequencies are responsible for what effects. This in itself is a dramatic step forward.

However, there remains at least one irresolvable topic even with this process. EEG responses are generally from around 8 Hz to, say, 100 Hz. Many of the ambient frequencies we are certain lie outside this band. Hence the question— can we detect and understand all health effects in crop circles? The answer is most likely no, but the use of this technology should offer further insights to enable us to broaden our diagnostic base.

9

THE OTHER SIDE
OF THE COIN:
NEGATIVE EFFECTS

If the only prayer you ever say in your entire life is thank you, it will be enough.

MEISTER ECKHART (1260–1328)

IN THIS CHAPTER WE WILL CONTINUE our human interaction journey and examine crop circle effects on the systemic system. Systemic circulation is the part of the cardiovascular system that carries oxygenated blood away from the heart to the body and returns deoxygenated blood back to the heart. This area of study includes the body as a whole, and we will be looking at such symptoms as dizziness, weak knees, leg pain, and other physical reactions as well as the gut effects of nausea, diarrhea, sudden hunger, and so forth.

I have found that I receive more negative than positive reports about visits to crop circles, as people generally expect to feel well and are surprised when they do not. Indeed they are more likely to remark on an ill effect, whereas if they feel better or happier than normal it is often attributed to other factors such as the beauty of the formation, the warm Sun, a day out, or being in the country with family or friends. It is not until there is a markedly noticeable feeling of well-being that the experience is described as being out of the ordinary.

Having visited over a hundred formations, I have personally experienced most of these different symptoms. My strong advice is that if you feel ill or uncomfortable in any way, leave the formation.

Once again we are looking at a multitude of reports so being selective is of the essence.

In 2007 an extraordinary formation appeared in East Field, Alton Barnes, near Marlborough, Wiltshire, a location that regularly hosts crop circles, and is an area of great electrical activity due to the complex pattern of energy lines running through the field together as well as the presence of underground aquifers. I received the following report:

THROWN DOWN WITH ALL HIS MIGHT

After lying down for about ten minutes, I proceeded to stand up, at which point, halfway up, I was strongly pulled backward to the ground, hitting my head and back very hard. As I was getting up, I felt and saw a circular motion around me like waves of energy going very fast, especially to the side on the right behind me. It took me a couple of days to find the words to describe how I felt. I felt I had become part of two magnets coming together.

When I wrote back suggesting that her symptoms sounded like a "drop attack" she replied, "I am not looking for an answer to what happened to me. Imagine being picked up by a very large wrestler and THROWN DOWN with all his might onto your back, then you have some sense of what happened."

A second event was described with similar effects. "I nearly went flying backward, only managing to save myself by grabbing big handfuls of wheat as I did not want to ruin the pattern by falling back onto the ground. After this I slowly tottered out leaning on a friend, back in one piece when outside the circle."

Could these experiences have been the result of an atonic seizure or drop attack? A drop attack is a seizure in which a person suddenly loses muscle tone and strength and, unless supported, falls down, also called a drop seizure. Atonic means a lack of muscle tone and strength due to uncontrolled electrical activity in the brain. Drop attacks are sudden spontaneous falls while standing or walking, with complete recovery in seconds or minutes. There is usually no recognized loss of consciousness, and the event is remembered. In most instances (64 percent), the cause of the drop attack is never definitively established.

As already explained, one day each summer I bring together as many

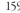

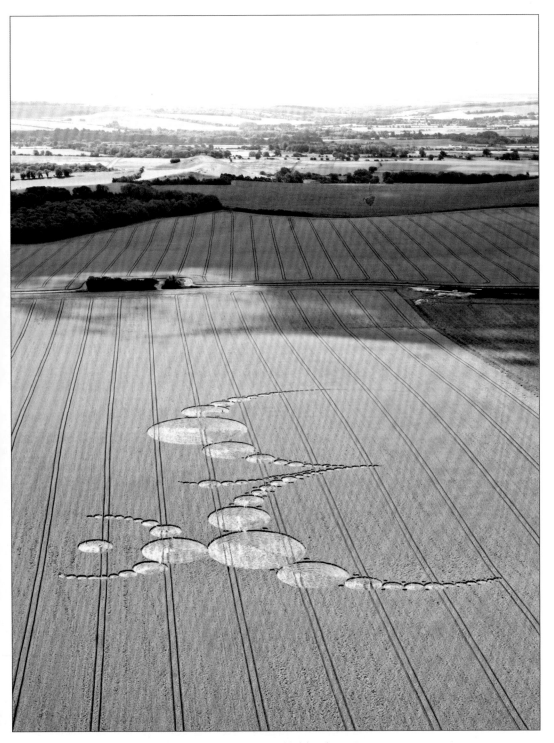

Fig. 9.1. 070707, East Field, Alton Barnes,
near Marlborough, Wiltshire, July 7, 2007.

scientists as possible using different techniques in order to try and establish a noticeable change between the control tests and the repeated tests conducted inside a crop circle. The 2007 East Field, Alton Barnes, formation was our chosen crop circle. Due to the number of bizarre effects reported, this formation is worthy of being singled out. These reports remain the most extraordinary and varied that I have ever received from one formation. The majority of them were negative despite initially starting off as positive.

I HAD HORRIBLE NIGHTMARES

The comments below are just some of the reports I received from our group.

- "I am not prone to nightmares, but had some horrible ones, probably for about two weeks afterward. I can't remember them now, but they were nasty and stayed with me all day, dreams of death, injury, and so forth."
- "I had a sore throat and sore eyes also for about two weeks."
- "I am not generally a moody person, quite laid back really, but felt very angry for a long time—probably a month or even more? I am a counselor, so am fairly self-aware, and again, am generally a positive person, not given to dwelling on negatives. I tried to find all sorts of explanations for why I felt so bad for so long, but there didn't seem to be any tangible reason."
- "I also had a disruption to my menstrual cycle."

Hazel Drummond, who had been with me in the small satellite circle after we had concluded the tests, ran around skipping like a schoolgirl. She had also lain flat on the ground. She reported that subsequently she suffered appalling nightmares (the type that are so terrible they wake one up in a muck sweat), panic attacks, and vibrating fingers for almost a week afterward. She also found it almost impossible to concentrate on her work.

Another member of the research group reported:

- "I've been very weary but not aching, and mentally unfocused, particularly yesterday where I got no work done . . . just pottering about and talking with people. Sleep has been very disrupted and unsatisfying. I woke this morning at 1:29 and never really got back into a deep sleep."

Anne Leonard, vice president of the Dowsing Society, financial adviser, and founder of Operation New World,* wrote telling me how she felt the following day.

- "Felt dizzy and dopey. I don't know how else to describe it but really the day floated by somehow. I had a letter to sign and send off and I WAS NOT ABLE TO DO IT."

I had not heard from Christopher Weeks, so I telephoned him on the Thursday after our visit. He told me that unlike the others he had wanted to get out of the circle almost as soon as he entered. His heart was thumping and he felt unwell. He told me that subsequently he had had "panic attacks, terrible dreams, depression," and his mind had been like "treacle." He had been unable to get on with his work.

THE PAIN WAS EXCRUCIATING

The night after our scientific tests, I woke at 1:20 a.m. with the most terrible pains running from inside my toes all the way up my shinbone to just under my knees. I tumbled out of bed and clung to the side of the bed for what seemed like an eternity. The pain was excruciating, and I did not know how long I was going to be able to cope with such a degree of agony. After approximately ten minutes the pain went, leaving a dull ache. I felt sure my legs would be covered in bruises the following morning, but to my amazement there was not a blemish to be seen. However my legs ached for the next five days. I am a crampy person but this was something quite different; my muscles were not in spasm. Also it seemed that the pain was located close to or in my shinbone.

My experience reminded me of a report sent in by someone who had entered the formation on the morning it had appeared and who had knelt down on the flattened crop.

I went into the formation 1:30 p.m. and had left the field itself by 2:30 p.m. Time of the first "spasm" to both legs: eight and a half hours later, lasting for about twenty minutes. Then there was a gap of about three-quarters of an hour and then I had another "spasm" on the right leg only, same area.

*www.opnewworld.co.uk.

First event: I was walking normally from a sofa in my living room toward my hall, when some twenty feet from the sofa, the sudden onset of pain forced me to the floor, due to the complete seizure of both legs. The pain was generated from beyond the toes to just below the knee, up the line of the shinbone. It was not in the muscles—all of which were quite relaxed during this experience. I am not a "crampy" person, and want it on record that this experience, while producing very acute physical responses—did NOT actually occur within the bone or leg itself. I also immediately knew that this was related to my earlier visit to the crop formation in East Field. So I waited it out, while testing my ability to stand up from time to time. As soon as it ended, I staggered into my kitchen and treated it by drinking cider vinegar with honey and hot water. The second attack to the right leg occurred after I had gone to bed. It was also unstoppable, even in trying to bend, tense, and straighten muscles—there was no way of stopping the pain, which again focused on the length of the shinbone. Again the muscles were completely relaxed. However, knowing that this was a crop event, I used my mind to control the pain, get out of bed, and go and get more cider vinegar, honey, and hot water. Although I had a lingering sensation in the area around and external to my right leg only—for several days after the event—it did not come back. Given that my events, occurring outside the physical body, do not concur with the actual physical symptoms of peroneal nerve problems, I am thus far of the conclusion that this event occurred in the etheric but was "picked up" by the sensors in the physical body. Perhaps surprisingly, I find myself grateful for the experience—it is still most educational!

In order to try to get a scientific explanation for my experience, I eventually went to see my doctor, who ruled out any vascular condition owing to the fact that my legs were not bruised. After such excruciating pain I could not believe that my legs did not show any evidence of my horrible experience.

She said I had described it as a nerve pain. We have a nerve called the peroneal that is associated with the sciatic nerve originating in the L5 lumbar vertebra. This nerve would act as a neurotransmitting agent, being triggered as a result of some unknown energy force, possibly electromagnetic. It would appear that the pain was the result of a change in the current transmitting through nerve cells.

Another member of the team told me that she had also been woken with terrible leg pains during the night following her visit and had been unable to get back to sleep.

A woman who on entry was as excited "as a schoolgirl all over again and full of life," went from one circle to the next, each one feeling different. She then

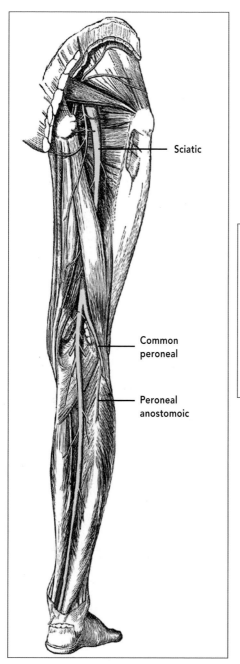

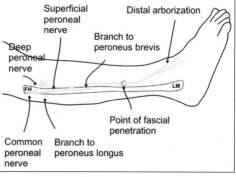

Fig. 9.2. Two illustrations showing the location of the peroneal nerve.

started to feel that everything was not OK, couldn't relax, and felt nauseous.

How can we explain this collection of independent experiences, a number of which lasted several days?

We are all surrounded by auras or electrical fields; the electrical field of our natural environment is known as the Schumann resonance, vibrating at frequencies ranging between 8 and 32 Hz. Evidence of extremely low frequencies (ELFs) is seen in hormonal activity, governed by the pituitary and pineal glands deep within our brains. However, not only are we experiencing exposure to this natural energy field but also the residual frequencies of the originating descending crop circle force. How our physical and emotional behavioral patterns are affected and how we react will vary considerably, as we are all individuals endowed with our own particular metabolic clock.

I STARTED BLACKING OUT

Centre of Crop Circle Studies* branch coordinator Carol Pederson visited a formation located at Whiskey Hill Road, near Hubbard, Oregon, with Keith Ardinger, and made a close examination of the laid crop. She sent me this excellent report.

When I first went in, I walked along the outer pathway and entered each circle as I came to it. Along the way, I felt dizzy several times. When we started to measure I began feeling a little sick but stuck with it. We started across one circle and reached the intersection of the northmost circle with its outer pathway, and I told Keith I wasn't feeling so well, and he told me to sit down for a while. I kept on and then started blacking out and really feeling sick. I knew if I stayed longer I would pass out completely. So I told him I had to leave the circle without completing the measuring and immediately (dizzily) picked up my bag and walked along the outer path out toward the weed field toward the van. I had an imperative need to get out of there quickly. This is all very peculiar because I am very thorough and NEVER give up my work until I am done, and yet

---

*The Centre for Crop Circle Studies was founded in England at Easter in 1990. It was the first academic society dedicated to the serious research of crop circles. I was a founder member. Later branches, under the banner of the United Kingdom mother branch, evolved all over the Western world. It finally dissolved in 2005. However certain overseas branches continued to operate and the story relating to one above was operating in the United States.

this time I just felt compelled to get out and fast. When I got to the van I put my head down on the hood and rested. I do not attribute this experience to the heat of the day; it was only 85 high that day, and it was about 5:30 anyway at that time. I am used to working in the heat; Keith and I spent about eight hours in 100-degree heat in Eltopia researching that formation, and I had just come back last week from Boise, Idaho, where I walked around a Basque Festival for three days in about 100-degree heat. So I attribute this experience to residual energy of the formation and that it affected me adversely.

Japanese author and crop circle researcher Maseo Maki took a group of his fellow countrymen into the Beckhampton "Knot" near Avebury, Wiltshire, in summer 1999. Later that evening, after having returned to their hotel in Marlborough, several of them suffered from severe nosebleeds. I understood that none of these sufferers was prone to nosebleeds and indeed did not suffer any further reoccurrence of the problem during the remainder of their tour. Epistaxis (nosebleed) is normally due to: (*a*) trauma/injury, (*b*) infection, (*c*) allergy, (*d*) malignant growths, (*e*) bleeding disorders.

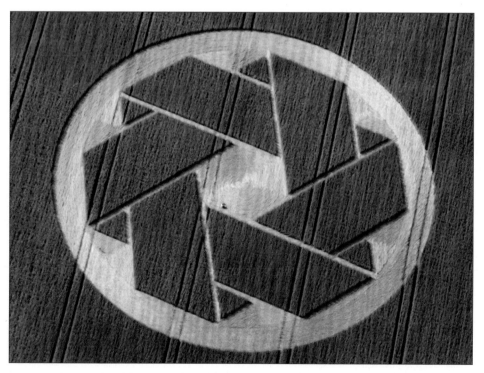

Fig. 9.3. Beckhampton Knot near Avebury, Wiltshire, July 28, 1999.

HUNT THE BOTTLE

Unfortunately, longtime friend and researcher Christopher Weeks is becoming more and more reluctant to come into crop circles with me.

On one particular occasion after we had visited the famous 2003 formation at Ogbourne St. George, north of Marlborough, to bury my bottles of water, Christopher developed severe gout within forty-eight hours. This is not the first time it has happened to him after visiting crop circles. His gout recovered, we returned a week later to collect the bottles, and all went well until I was digging up the final pair of controls when I noticed something unusual. "You have buried them one on top of each other instead of side by side." "Yes," said Christopher. As I removed the first bottle Christopher said he would dig out the second and took my trowel. We were chatting, and it was several moments before Christopher said the other bottle was no longer there! No longer there? That was impossible, we had both seen it, and indeed I had remarked on the white bottle top and the curious way Christopher had buried the pair! Christopher was so disturbed by its disappearance that he set about digging up the area with furious determination. I feared he might excavate the entire perimeter of the field. The bottle was never found. Into what dimension had it disappeared?

Within forty-eight hours Christopher developed gout once more. We know that gout occurs as result of uric acid crystals collecting around joints, causing painful inflammation. It is sometimes thought that an abundance of rich food and red wine or port can be the cause. Christopher is a vegetarian and teetotaler who eats mainly organic foods.

RED WINE AND CHOCOLATES

Three other people who visited the formation all felt extremely thirsty as they left. Instead of drinking the water they had brought with them, they all craved red wine. Two of them had forgotten this effect when they revisited the formation at a later date. Unexpectedly this effect was repeated. They are naturally moderate red-wine drinkers but this compulsion was something different. Could there be a chemical constituent that is common to both red wine and the cause of gout? Relating to red-wine reports, it has been suggested to me that the exogenous stimulus was a "kick" to the reward centers of the brain, rather than a subconscious seeking of an ingredient. This brings us to (*a*) dopamine production overstimulation, (*b*) the orbitofrontal cortex behind the eyes, and

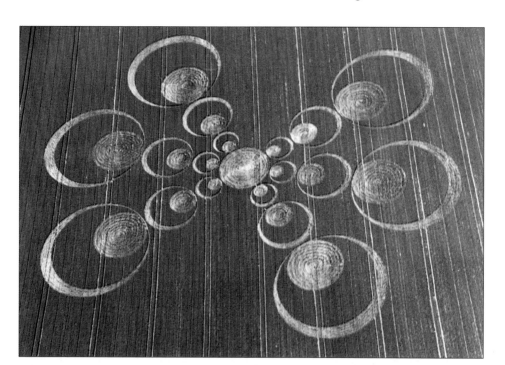

Fig. 9.4. Ogbourne St. George, north of Marlborough, Wiltshire, June 15, 2003.

(c) opioid stimulation (endorphins and enkephalins) and the ventral pallidum.

The next question is the energy input. Eddy currents, produced when magnetic fields traverse the brain, are now coming to the fore in physics.

Several years ago a young man sent me a report telling me that despite feeling slightly nauseous while inside a formation, he had desperately craved chocolate. Many people suffer from this condition, the late Princess Diana included. We are told that whereas chocolate craving is often linked to eating disorders, there are other possible reasons. The main active ingredient of chocolate is cocoa, a significant source of the stimulant theobromine, which is a known mood elevator.

In tests it has been shown that alcohol-loving rats, given the choice, will actually replace their alcohol intake in preference of chocolate. By doing this, the rats increase their level of dopamine, as chocolate appears to stimulate its production. A study of rats shows that dopamine kick-starts a brain messenger chemical called DARPP-32 that in turn activates hormones that make females interested in sex—hence Valentine's Day chocolates.

Researchers at the Neurosciences Institute in San Diego have also discovered that novel constituents in cocoa powder and chocolate are chemical cousins of anandamide, which binds to the same brain receptor sites as marijuana.

This means that chocolate chemicals may activate receptors for marijuana and thus mimic its psychoactive effects of heightened sensations and euphoria.

What are the reasons for these strange cravings? Is there a dopamine link between chocolate and red wine? But what about gout? When dealing with complex subtle energies, their effects on areas of the brain are still not fully understood.

DYING FOR A DRINK AND AS HUNGRY AS A HORSE

Once again we must consider the hypothalamus, as it regulates our body fluids and appetite.

The author and researcher Freddy Silva reported:

About half a mile before reaching the formation I felt pressure on my chest. In the formation I felt pressure near my pineal gland, also disorientation and massive dehydration.

In addition he had a severe headache. On leaving the formation he drank six pints of water within the next hour. The extreme thirst lasted for twelve hours.

After I'd been in the crop formation for about twenty minutes I became aware that I was feeling very shaky (especially my legs) and I was incredibly hungry. I nearly tore open my sandwich box on the spot. The feeling lasted for the remainder of the day.

On many occasions effects take people by surprise, as in my case. I am not a big eater and quite often go comfortably without food from a light breakfast until a late lunch maybe around 4:00 p.m. We had just finished a good lunch at the normal time, before visiting the Butser Hill formation, near Petersfield, Hampshire, to conduct hormone tests. The acute hunger I experienced as I walked out of the circle was therefore most surprising and out of the ordinary.

MY SHOES KEPT FALLING OFF

Arthritis and rheumatism sufferers seem to gain noticeable but temporary relief. Longtime sufferer Leslie Clementson has, over the years, sent me very interesting reports on her experiences in formations (see pages 1–2).

The effects seem to vary from circle to circle. However, in some formations such as the Lockeridge event (figs. 3.3 and 3.4), her swollen feet were so improved that her shoes kept falling off. The positive effects were, unfortunately, only temporary.

We need to examine the possible reason for these encouraging reactions. We do not know enough about the "cause" of rheumatism or arthritis, but we do know the effect is inflammation. Could the residual effects of the electromagnetic fields present in some formations be acting as an anti-inflammatory? We are told that there are over a hundred types of arthritis, including osteoarthritis and gout. The word *arthritis* means "joint inflammation." Inflammation is one of the body's natural reactions to disease or injury, and includes swelling, pain, and stiffness. Inflammation that lasts for a very long time or recurs, as in arthritis, can lead to tissue damage.

Rheumatoid arthritis is an autoimmune disease. With rheumatoid arthritis, something seems to trigger the immune system to attack the joints and sometimes other organs of the body. The exact cause of rheumatoid arthritis is unknown, but it is thought to be due to a combination of genetic, environmental, and hormonal factors. Other theories suggest that a virus or bacteria may alter the immune system, causing it to attack the joints.

COLD HANDS AND HOT FEET

Other bizarre reports come trickling in. Interior designer Polly Blackett sent me a report after visiting a formation the day it appeared. She was with a group from London.

> I got the usual sort of connection, which I get with all formations of one sort or another. My fingers went numb and I almost lost consciousness I was so cold and only just thawed out when I borrowed someone's extra jacket and ate everybody's food and after the driver put the heating up full blast for about an hour on our way back to London. The last time I remember being so cold was about twenty years ago when I went white-water rafting in Colorado and had my foot in ice all day.

Polly mentioned that she had fallen on pavement earlier that week and had trapped a nerve but that this had healed by the time she entered the formation. None of the others in the group experienced anything unusual.

The hypothalamus is a very important part of the forebrain; it lies below the thalamus and forms the lower part of the ventricle and its floor. Its integrity is essential to life, for it is concerned with the "vegetative" functions. It plays a major part in regulating the temperature of the body, body weight and appetite, sexual behavior and rhythms, blood pressure, and fluid balance, and can even be said to be the physical basis of the emotions.

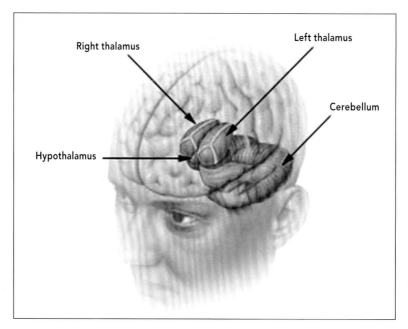

Fig. 9.5. The hypothalamus. Many of the effects from crop circles experienced by people are a result of activity in the hypothalamus.

CLEARING THE HEAD?

There are numerous reports from hay-fever sufferers such as one visiting a circle for the first time. She was nervous about going into the 1998 "Beltane Wheel" circle near Silbury Hill as it was in oilseed rape (canola), a plant to which she was allergic. However she plucked up courage and decided to brave it.

"I felt pleasantly light-headed the whole time; my sinuses cleared." I mentioned this to my companion, and a young man overheard me and said his sinuses had dried up too. Another man suffering from hay fever found that

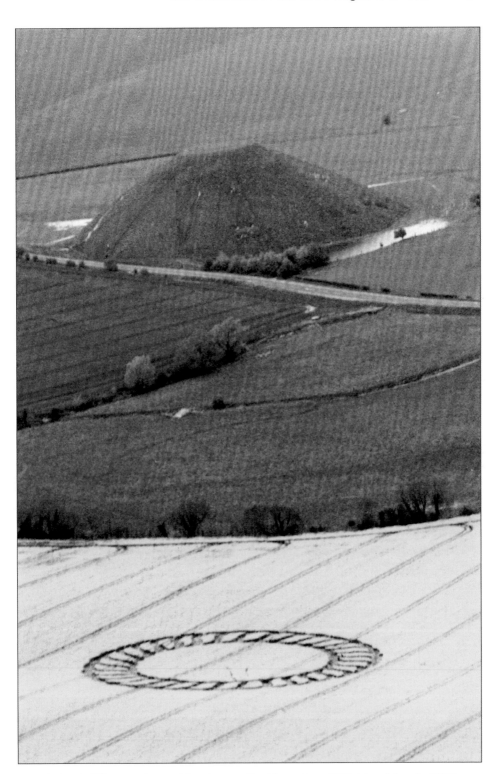

Fig. 9.6. Silbury Beltane Wheel, near Beckhampton, Wiltshire, May 4, 1998.

whereas he had been "streaming on entering the formation" he dried up during his visit.

She was in the formation for some time and felt her throat getting quite constricted, despite trying not to breathe in the pollen. Her throat was sore when she got home and remained congested for several days. It then cleared and she has not suffered from hay fever since.

A few days later she also went into the Silbury "Scorpion" in the adjoining field, and as she was walking in it her fingertips felt as if they were being burnt by a cigarette or something similar, an intensely hot feeling. She felt so strange she had to come out.

Hay fever symptoms are caused when a person has an allergic reaction to pollen.

Pollen is a fine powder released by plants as part of their reproductive cycle. Pollen contains proteins that can cause the nose, eyes, throat, and sinuses (small air-filled cavities behind your cheekbones and forehead) to become swollen, irritated, and inflamed.

To alleviate these symptoms antihistamine is prescribed. Antihistamines work by blocking the effects of a protein called histamine. They're available in tablet or capsule form (oral antihistamines), creams, lotions, and gels (topical antihistamines) and as a nasal spray.

We are told that "histamine is a protein that the immune system uses to help protect the body's cells against infection." The immune system is the body's natural defense against illness and infection.*

If the immune system detects a harmful foreign object, such as bacteria or a virus, it will release histamine into nearby cells. The histamine causes small blood vessels to expand and the surrounding skin to swell. This is known as inflammation.

The expansion of the blood vessels allows an increased number of infection-fighting white blood cells to be sent to the site of the infection. The swelling of the surrounding skin also makes it harder for an infection to spread to other parts of the body.

Histamine is usually a useful protein, but if you're having an allergic reaction it's sometimes necessary to block its effects. Allergic reactions occur when your immune system mistakes a harmless substance, such as pollen, as a threat. The release of histamine causes the process of inflammation to begin and leads

---

*See http://en.wikipedia.org/wiki/Histamine.

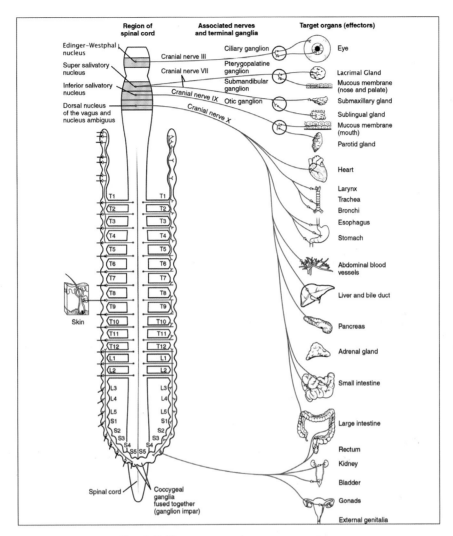

Fig. 9.7. The autonomic nervous system.

to nearby tissue becoming red and swollen. It can also affect the nerves in the skin, making the skin feel itchy.

Could the crop circles be acting as antihistamines? I believe that once more we are looking to the hypothalamus. The hypothalamus is also responsible for the autonomic nervous system (ANS) that affects involuntary conditions such as heart rate, digestion, respiratory rate, salivation, and perspiration.

There is a consciousness present in everything around us, the "Gaia" consciousness as described by professor James Lovelock, and in genuine formations, due to their very size and complexity, there is evidence of an additional intelligence, intent, and focusing.

ANNE LEONARD'S ADVENTURE

Pending receiving the scientific results, I have to tell you that, unusually for me, I found the time spent in the Silbury Hill formation to be wildly beneficial! This is a teeny bit surprising given the journey back home! A friend had very kindly agreed to give me a lift to Guildford, whence he was bound anyway, offering to drop me off at the railway station, which was on his route home. A happy arrangement. Picture my surprise therefore to find him driving into Terminal 1 at Heathrow!

On reaching Terminal 1, to my surprise, we suddenly shot left, straight down a 45-degree slope, not, I think, open normally to the public. This was a sort of semi-vertical cul-de-sac. There was, however, a sharp bend [90 degrees] round which, undaunted, our driver swung his car scraping through a most narrow passage, thereby entering a car park from the wrong end. Coming eventually to a barrier, an attendant appeared shouting what the hell did we think we were doing and this barrier was to let people in, from the other side, and was not for letting anyone out! How had we got in? he cried. Again, undaunted, my friend informed the varlet he was to LET US OUT whereupon the pole was raised and out we scudded. Hours later, as I think I told you, we stopped at a hitherto unknown (to me) railway station where, said my friend, "trains might be going to London." I still couldn't tell you the name of the place. It looked deserted. But eventually a train did come along and amazingly took me to London and this was free of charge for there was nobody to pay.

Dear, dear. I think I was blessed to get home at all!

The feel-good factor is terrific, my energy levels have soared and, most striking of all, I have suddenly lost weight! Several pounds in fact!

(Possibly the journey helped!!!)

Love from Anne

ROCKLEY MANOR: LUCY DISAPPEARS

A personal experience occurred after conducting a scientific test in the 1999 Rockley formation at Hackpen just below the chalk White Horse. Control tests were to be carried out at Rockley Manor with kind permission of the owners Richard and Fiona North.

I led the way in my car with the scientists following in their car. At the

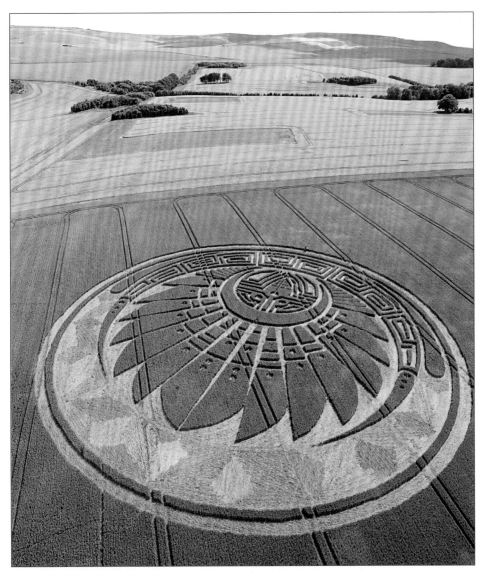

Fig. 9.8. Opposite Silbury Hill, near Beckhampton, Wiltshire, July 5, 2009.
A formation with arcs and graduated segments, resembling a Greek key pattern.

Rockley signpost we turned off, and on my right were two splendid stone entrance pillars beyond which was a long curving driveway with parkland on either side, leading to a lovely white Georgian house. Being uncertain if this was Rockley Manor, I continued down the lane with the stone wall on my right until coming to a side entrance with two stone posts. As there were no other houses about, clearly this was Rockley Manor.

I got out of my car and walked back to the scientists who had drawn up behind me and told them I was going to turn round and go back and drive down the front entrance. They said they would follow me. I backed my car into a small lane in front of the scientists' car. I then changed my mind and decided to drive in via the side entrance. Consequently I drove right across and in front of the car behind me and expected them to follow.

When I reached the house, Fiona's charming mother, Lili Millais, came out to greet me. "I am so sorry," I said, "I have come in the wrong way. I meant to drive down the front entrance at the top of the lane."

Lili looked at me strangely and said, "But this is the front entrance; there has not been a front entrance at the top of the lane for well over one hundred years!"

Where were the scientists? At last they arrived hot and bothered. "Where on earth did you go, Lucy, you completely disappeared?"

I could not possibly have disappeared as I had been right in front of them all the time I had been in the lane. Also they were scientists with rational, logical brains so it seems unlikely they should be victims of over active imaginations or self-delusion.

So what is the answer? Where had I gone? Just as I had regressed in time when seeing the front drive, could my disappearance be explained by my entry into another earlier time and place?

This apparent lapse of time and space has happened to me on several occasions and seems quite normal at the time. Also on this occasion I could see the scientists at all times until turning into the side entrance when they were hidden from my view by the wall. Maybe I had inadvertently resonated to the same frequency as the events of that time and had thus entered another time dimension taking my car with me. Rather like Doctor Who and the Tardis!

When I asked the scientists for their version of events, they said. "You simply disappeared; you were there one moment and gone the next. We drove back down the lane expecting to find you at any moment. We searched everywhere."

On a similar vein a bizarre event happened to Ron Russell, a long-time friend and crop circle researcher and enthusiast.

RON RUSSELL'S AVEBURY STORY

John and I went into the "Nested Scorpion" at Avebury Trusloe about 11.30 p.m. on August 11, 1994, the day of its arrival. I was fortunate to fly that day and got some excellent photos of it, but we had a lot of stuff to do, and we couldn't visit it until that night. It was easy to find, and we carefully made our way into it along the tramlines. I was delighted with the energy I felt. There was a tingling in my feet and legs, and I was about to bliss out. We walked a short way into it, and John wanted to meditate, but curiously I did not and conceived of a plan to take flash photos of the centres of the circles, which I proceeded to do, until I ran out of film. "Oh darn," I thought, "now I'll have to go back to the car." I sent John a strong telepathic message about what I was up to and went out of the formation to get some more film. I retraced our path toward the edge of the field. I walked and walked and walked but I never found the edge of the field, and I became concerned as so much time was passing. I trudged onward knowing that the edge was near (it must be, surely) and the grass grew shorter and the tramlines disappeared and I found myself in a state of disbelief. I looked hard every which way and spotted some flickering lights in the distance, which I trudged towards, sweating as a result of this long walk, which I estimated to have been about thirty minutes.

As I approached the flickering lights and some intervening bushes, I could see they were fires. I stopped in my tracks and thought to myself, "They don't have open fires in Avebury Trusloe at this time of night. What has happened to me? Have I gone into some sort of dimensional shift here? And what about the tramlines disappearing? And the air becoming somehow thicker?" I was a bit alarmed and wished that John were closer so I could investigate this with some more safety, like a buddy system. I slowly walked closer to the bushes, and I could clearly see on the other side there were two bonfires and several short people milling about them in a sort of a little clearing surrounded by several thatched huts. "What a great opportunity!" I thought. And as I was about to approach this scene the thought of being burned at the stake flashed through my mind, and I paused to consider this. "What if I have slipped over to the fifteenth century?" I asked myself. "If I enter their world what are they going to think of me? I doubt if I would be invited to dinner. This was not a very open period in men's thoughts and beliefs and with my clothing and mannerisms and cameras slung around my neck (without film!) I would guess they would think poorly of me and might harm me as I did not fit into their world."

Slowly I backtracked to get John and enact the buddy system. I followed my tracks through the short wheat and finally came to the faint beginnings of the tramlines I had come down. I followed this for about thirty minutes

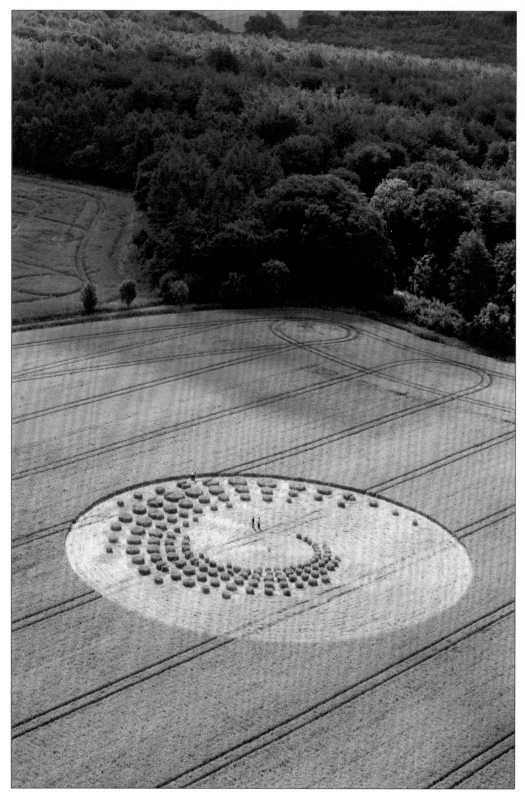

Fig. 9.9. Forest Farm, near Marlborough, Wiltshire, July 16, 2014.

and at last found my way back into the formation where John was standing. "Come with me, John!" I exclaimed. "I have found a time door," and we proceeded back the way I had just come except that we came right away to the edge of the field and the car! As I explained all this to him and apologised for my long absence, which I calculated at over an hour (I did not have my watch on), he looked at me in a bemused way and said, "Ron, you've only been gone five minutes!" I was stunned and thought he was jesting with me and went over all the details again. He said that he had gotten my message and that he had finished his meditation and had just gotten up when I returned, which had been about five minutes! We could never locate the encampment with the fire. Was I delusional? I thought not, but am at a loss to explain this further.

This experience seems to be one more instance of accessing another space, time, and dimension by subconsciously tuning into the same vibrational frequency as the event.

There is also a story told by John from Harlow. He managed to interest a farmer who took him to a formation on his land and told him to go in. As the farmer stood by the edge of the formation, John asked him if he was coming in too.

"No," he replied. "I am not going in there again. Every time I have been in I have needed sixteen hours of sleep." Sixteen hours of sleep is more than any farmer can afford, especially at harvest time!

MY TEETH WENT ON EDGE

Both Christopher and his daughter Emily had adverse experiences in the Forest Farm formation, near Marlborough. Christopher told me that

entering the field all felt still and calm as did the approach to the circle when within about ten feet of the circle it felt like pushing through mud or walking through the outer shell of the circle. Once inside to me it felt like being in a void. I was unable to distinguish any particular parts of the circle from another, but when near the edge there definitely felt to be a lot of energy in a way that I have not come across before. While in the circle two of my teeth went on edge and it felt as if current was passing between the two of them; this passed when I exited the circle and has not recurred since.

As an aside, while in the circle I shut my eyes and let any other information flood into my head; this is not generally a good move but all that came through was that that field would be better suited to cows! I was aware of much more energy going on outside the circle than in it.

I was aware that Emily wasn't feeling well where she was lying just inside the perimeter so I dowsed for a more beneficial spot. Emily writes:

When I walked into the circle it felt muted and very sheltered, even though the field wasn't sheltered at all.

Once we were inside the circle I felt quite dizzy, and it felt like my legs weren't connected to the rest of my body. The left-hand side of the circle made me feel nauseous and dizzy when I went in it. On a certain spot in the circle I disappeared from any dowsing.

On hearing this James Lyons dowsed the area where Emily had entered. There appeared to be a void (torsion field?) at that exact point.

When I was leaving the circle, I felt much better than when in the circle, but I could feel certain sections on the outside of the circle where it felt like my nose was being pinched then released on one side.

COMMENTS BY JAMES LYONS

In considering health effects in crop circles, we have in particular the problem of trying to explain possible mechanisms, which could account for the very significant spectrum of effects on individuals. Although crop circles have acquired a degree of notoriety in this respect, it has to be stated that stone circles and ancient sites have a long-standing reported history of producing health-related phenomena.

We have consistently emphasized that the whole of the Cosmos is electrical in nature. The most prolific subatomic particles are the proton and the electron. These are the two building blocks of the most common gas in the Cosmos, namely Hydrogen. On Earth, they combine to create the gas we are familiar with. We know that it is lighter than air from its former use in children's balloons.

Outside the immediate atmosphere of the Earth, the protons and electrons exist in all space in their dissociated form. It is termed the plasma state. The plasma, or fourth, state of matter is by far the most common state, more common than the other three more familiar states of solid, liquid, and gas. Weather phenomena on Earth, such as lightning and tornadoes, reveal most clearly this plasma state. Both have significant effects on electrical apparatus.

It is now known, but far from accepted, that our Sun is a ball of plasma, sending electric current streams to Earth and, indeed, to all objects in our Solar System.

We know that the grid network of spiraling filaments in space is mimicked within the Earth, creating the grid of energy lines on which all medieval churches and ancient sites were built. We have discussed the colloquially termed spider's web patterns or acupuncture points on the Earth. These are the "graph paper" on which crop circles form. Not surprisingly, when crop circles are formed there remains a swirling cloud of dissociated air. It is a mixture of protons, electrons, and indeed nitrogen, which combines with the air to form nitrates in the crop. Potentially, nitrogen dioxide could also be formed, which is the pollution component of diesel engines. This, to our knowledge, has never been measured.

We turn to the effects of this electrically charged local environment on living matter. We have identified the beneficial effects on humans, but what about the downside? It is well known that in certain stone circles there exist fertility stones upon which aspiring mothers will remain seated for some time. We know from hormone testing in crop circles that substances such as estrogen are created and pass through the root chakra up the cross-wound spinal cord into the hypothalamus and on to appropriate receptors.

This effect does not have to be necessarily in stone or crop circles. Some time ago, the media publicized the famous checkout desk in a Warrington supermarket at which ladies wishing to become pregnant were advised to sit because there seemed to be an electrically-charged environment at that location. From afar, it is clear that, unbeknown to the management, there simply had to be a narrow columnar vortex beneath the appropriate cash desk. Its energy-spiraling properties were such that it imitated the fertility stone-circle effects.

Not surprisingly, there is a downside to crop circle energies. To initiate a discussion of this aspect of crop circle energies, it might be beneficial to say a little about some science that acquired a large degree of notoriety. We turn to one Wilhelm Reich, a medical doctor and psychoanalyst from the first half of the twentieth century.

In addition to his psychological writings, he also developed a theory of human health based on his discovery of what he called *Orgone*. The word derives from organism and orgasm! In simple terms it is a way of generating, in a so-called accumulator, techniques for supposedly curing many conditions, including cancer. However, a version of this device emitted what was called DOR—Deadly Orgone. This proved to have in many cases deleterious effects on patients. Reich ended up in prison as a result his work.

DOR is prepared as a state of water. Dowsing the auric field of water in the DOR state immediately indicates its very small auric field. It is, in fact, drawing subtle energy, life force, or whatever term one prefers, from the body. This type of energy spiraling into the body is termed entropic since it draws the life force from the body.

In crop circles, there is a basic balanced energy field in most settled conditions. It emerges from the energy-pattern structure that creates the basic circle. Appendix 8 describes all this in some detail, but here we only need to note the fundamental process. From the top of the hemisphere covering a crop circle there is a nodal point, akin to a pole of a magnet. Needless to say, there is a complementary energy structure below. This is the status quo.

However, when a crop circle is being formed, this basic biconical energy field does not have its final geometrical form. It tends to have a very low "slope" angle to this virtual energy pyramid. We now understand that all living matter is far from resonant with this geometry. In fact, the geometry involved conditions the local space within the crop circle to such an extent that the vortex field motion has rotational frequencies so out of tune with normality that physical forces can emerge. Thus crop circle visitors can literally feel the effects of the rotating force field and, as we have seen on occasions, be thrown to the ground. It is somewhat analogous to being inside an electric motor!

Thus, to summarize the bad effects, we have to recognize that crop circles are the result of strong physical forces. Depending on when a crop circle is visited, the remnant electric field can still retain some of its "motor," and its characteristics are still present.

10

HISTORY AND
FORMATION THEORY

*Men are disturbed not by things that happen, but by their opinion
of the things that happen.*

Epictetus, Grecian Philosopher (55–135 CE)

WHEN WE TALK ABOUT THE HISTORY of crop circles, despite the general view that this is a modern phenomenon, we find ourselves taking a journey into the distant past, to the times of our ancestors.

Just as many artists painted small, almost unnoticed images of UFOs in their works, such as *The Annunciation,* Carlo Crevelli 1486 (National Gallery), or described an event, dating back to 776 in France, in the twelfth-century manuscript *Annales Laurissenses,* so did our forebears use whatever means they had on hand to record what they were actually witnessing in their lives; these records went unnoticed until recently.

This investigation leads to the wonderfully ancient and stylized Aboriginal cave drawings. These cave paintings were unknown to the Western world until discovered by Joseph Bradshaw in 1981 in an overhanging rock shelter facing the Roe River in Western Australia. Joseph Bradshaw was the first European to describe this style of Aboriginal art. These figures are known to the Ngarinyin Aboriginals as Gwion Gwion. Thousands of such cave drawings are to be found in the Kimberley area. The stylized drawing, sketched by Bradshaw, reveals people wearing strange headgear standing near a circular indentation on the ground (a crop circle?), with a kangaroo and a snake shown fleeing the scene in terror.

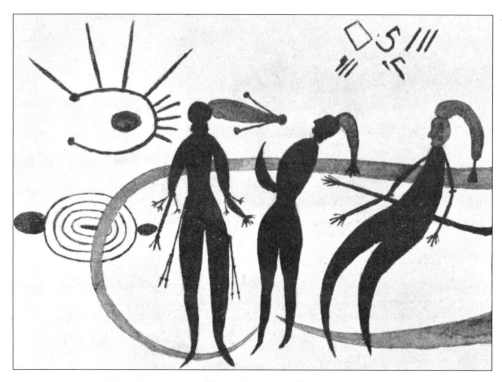

Fig. 10.1. A scene from the Australian cave paintings
discovered by Joseph Bradshaw in 1981.

Zulu holy man Credo Mutwa tells us that there have been equally ancient circles in Africa dating back some 4,000 years or more in certain arable fields of corn or millet that were considered sacred by the elders. The crop from these fields was never allowed to be cut but left as food for the birds.

Our investigation takes us to the connections between crop circles, stone circles, Pythagoras (427–347 BC), and the 11,000-year-old Göbekli temple in Turkey.

Six miles from Urfa, an ancient city in southeastern Turkey, Klaus Schmidt made one of the most startling archaeological discoveries of our time: massive carved stones about 11,000 years old, crafted and arranged by prehistoric people who had not yet developed metal tools or even pottery. The megaliths predate Stonehenge by some 6,000 years. The place is called Göbekli Tepe, and Schmidt, a German archaeologist who has been working there for more than a decade, is convinced it's the site of the world's oldest temple. The geometry found in the construction of this ancient temple mirrors the geometry we find in the crop circles.

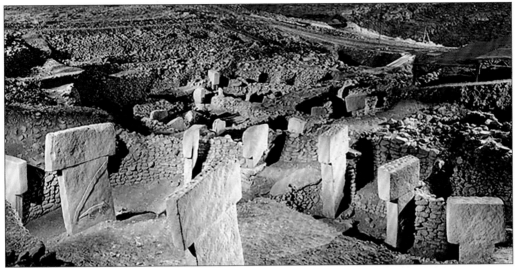

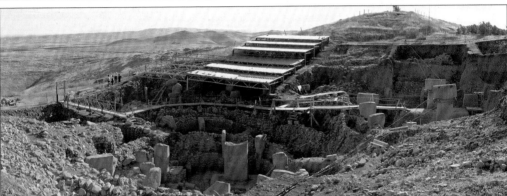

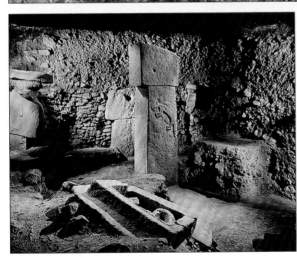

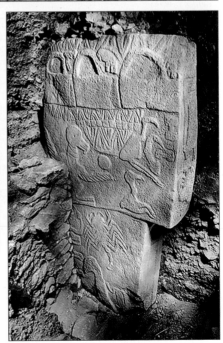

Fig. 10.2. The Göbekli Tepe Temple.

More evidence can be found at Newgrange in County Meath, on the eastern side of Ireland, which was built around 3200 BCE, during the Neolithic period, particularly the assortment of spiral and circular carvings on the kerbstone there. Indeed some of the carvings resemble the crop circles found in the fields in the early 1990s.

There is no overall consensus regarding the use of the site, but it has been speculated that it had some form of religious significance due to the fact that it is aligned with the rising Sun, which floods the stone room with light on the Winter Solstice. Carbon dating revealed that Newgrange monument is older than Stonehenge and the Great Pyramids of Giza. Was it a tomb?

Excavations have revealed deposits of both burnt and unburnt human bone in the passage, indicating human corpses were indeed placed within it, some of which had been cremated.

Moving forward in time we discover that in his book *Hypomnemata Antiquaria,* seventeenth-century antiquarian, historian, and philosopher John Aubrey (March 12, 1626–June 7, 1697)—after whom the Aubrey stones at Stonehenge are named—was perplexed by green grass circles on the Downs in Wiltshire. He wrote, "I presume they are generated from the breathing out of a fertile subterraneous vapour." He further wrote that "every tobacco-taker knows that 'tis no strange thing for a circle of smoke to be whiff'd out of the bowle of the pipe; but 'tis donne by chance."

Professor Robert Plot published a book entitled *A Natural History of Staffordshire* in 1686. In it he makes brief references to rings, circles, and other shapes found in grassy fields. Despite the detail of his writing there is uncertainty as to whether he was describing rings of fungi, known as faery rings, or genuine crop circles.

The 1678 woodcut of the Mowing Devil (fig. 10.3) is probably the most famous recorded crop circle event of early times. It shows a devil-like person cutting the crop with a scythe. The story behind this woodcut tells us of a farmer who, having rejected the price charged by a harvester, stormed off saying he would rather let the devil takes his oats. That night he heard strange sounds and saw strange lights, only to find on entering his field the following morning that his crop had been cut in round circles, frightening him to such a degree that he took to his heels and fled. It is thanks to the extensive research conducted by author Andy Thomas that we know about this story as he found and read the original—and now somewhat fragile—pamphlet in the British Library.

The Mowing-Devil:
Or, Strange NEWS out of
Hartford-ſhire.

Being a True Relation of a Farmer, who Bargaining with a Poor *Mower*, about the Cutting down Three Half Acres of *Oats*; upon the *Mower*'s asking too much, the *Farmer* ſwore, *That the Devil ſhould Mow it, rather than He*: And ſo it fell out, that that very Night, the Crop of *Oats* ſhew'd as if it had been all of a Flame; but next Morning appear'd ſo neatly Mow'd by the Devil, or ſome Infernal Spirit, that no Mortal Man was able to do the like.
Alſo, How the ſaid *Oats* ly now in the Field, and the Owner has not Power to fetch them away.

Licenſed, *Auguſt* 22th. 1678.

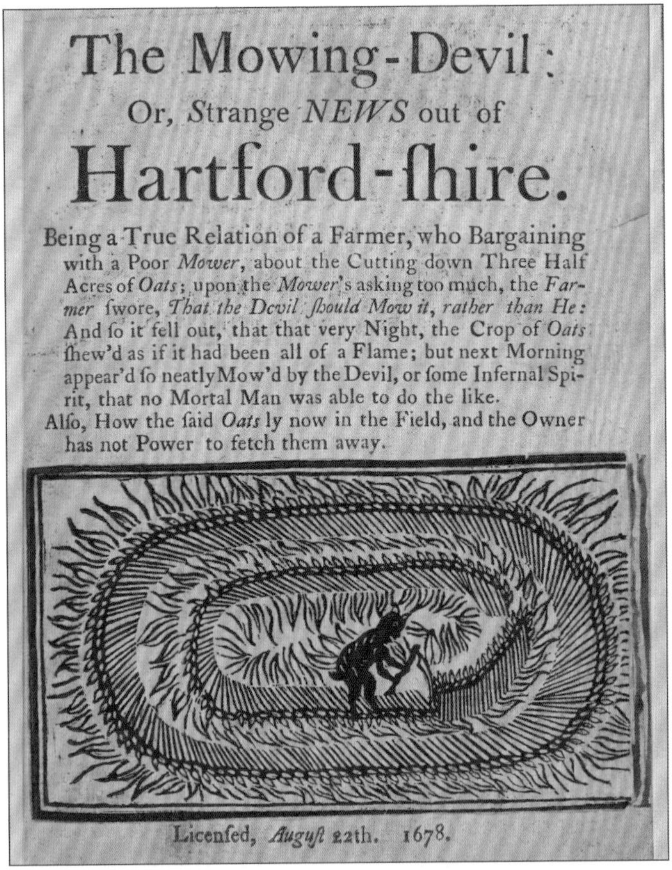

Fig. 10.3. A woodcut depicting a crop circle (later known as the Mowing Devil) from a publication in 1678.

Clearly this was of such importance that it was recorded, and that record has passed down to us through the ages.

During the course of the sixteenth century, King Henry VIII became interested in the customs of rural England and sent his antiquary, John Leland, on a fact-finding tour. In the course of this tour Leland asked the people of Wessex about their village-green ring dances.

"They are so intricate," he said. "How on Earth do you devise such complex routines?"

"We base them," came the reply, "on the magic grass designs that appear in our fields."

Bringing us closer to modern times is a report from July 1880 by John Capron (1829–1888), an amateur astronomer and highly respected spectroscopist. He discovered the circles at the Hog's Back near Guildford, Surrey.

The *Surrey Advertiser* reported his findings at the time and many years later they were published in the respected scientific journal *Nature* in 1880 and reprinted in the January 2000 issue of the *Journal of Meteorology* (ISSN 0307–5966: Volume 25, pp. 20–21: "A case of genuine crop circles dating from July 1880—as published in *Nature* in the year 1880").

> The storms about this part of Surrey have been lately local and violent, and the effects produced in some instances curious. Visiting a neighbour's farm on Wednesday evening (21st), we found a field of standing wheat considerably knocked about, not as an entirety, but in patches forming, as viewed from a distance, circular spots.
>
> Examined more closely, these all presented much the same character, viz., a few standing stalks as a center, some prostrate stalks with their heads arranged pretty evenly in a direction forming a circle round the center, and outside these a circular wall of stalks, which had not suffered, I sent a sketch made on the spot, giving an idea of the most perfect of these patches. The soil is a sandy loam upon the greensand, and the crop is vigorous, with strong stems, and I could not trace locally any circumstances accounting for the peculiar forms of the patches in the field, nor indicating whether it was wind or rain, or both combined, which had caused them, beyond the general evidence everywhere of heavy rainfall. They were suggestive to me of some cyclonic wind action, and may perhaps have been noticed elsewhere by some of your readers.

In the 1930s, crop marks are mentioned twice in *Sussex Notes and Queries,* the journal of the Sussex Archeological Society.

In August 1932 it was reported that three dark rings about 40 yards in diameter and part of a fourth had been noted in barley on the lower southern slope of Stoughton Down near Chichester.

In October 1936 a lecturer on "Archeology from the Air" suggested crop marks noted that year could be indicative of ploughed out ditches of large barrows. He looked forward to other sites being revealed by aerial photography.

Several pilots during World War II reported flying over crop circles in the south of England. These were investigated by M15 fearing that they might be codes left for German pilots.

In 1963 a strange crater appeared in a field in Wiltshire that puzzled renowned astronomer Sir Patrick Moore. He attributed the crater to be of possible meteoric origin and sent a comprehensive report to *New Scientist* on August 8, 1963, which alerted both the press and the public.

In describing his inspection of the crater, Moore incidentally mentions several unusual circles of flattened wheat in fields adjoining the potato field in which the crater had appeared. At this time the term "crop circle" had not been coined, and there was no real public interest in crop circles as such; however, there can be little doubt that Moore was describing crop circles.

UFO NESTS

Australia too has had its circles. In 1974 there was a report of a circle measuring around twenty feet in diameter, which was discovered in a large field of saffron thistles in the Goolagong area in the Bathhurst District.

Diana Kearns, who sent me this story, had been awarded a grant by the Australian Film Commission; she was studying the possible correlation between UFOs and grid patterns/systems, ancient Aboriginal stone rows or stone circles in the UK, connected with the ley line system.

Just before Christmas 1974, she was telephoned by the UFO Society regarding this circle (or UFO nest as they are called in Australia). In Australia distances of up to two hundred miles are considered close by, so off she hurtled and was met by the farmer, Viv Huckel.

The field of thistles had been plowed up at the request of the Australian Broadcasting Commission, which made it a considerably less painful journey for Diana. "These thistles are as thick as the hair on a dog's back!"

The farmer, Viv Huckel, recounts:

What hit me when I first saw it was that it was very similar to nests found in the sugarcane beds up in Queensland. I drove around, finished plowing and came back and had another squizz at it. What intrigued me was that the center portion (about four foot across) was almost completely bare, and after that you started getting little stumps of saffron thistles—they'd been shredded. The further you got to the perimeter, pieces of stalk were just broken up; but the last couple of feet of thistles—and these are two feet high minimum—were completely knocked down in an anticlockwise direction, twisted up, and some had been torn out by the roots. It's pretty hard to pull a green saffron thistle out by the roots, mate!

The theory that animals might have squashed down the thistles was discounted by Viv, who had only had five head of cattle in that paddock in the previous six months.

"Like their female counterparts in the human race, they like their creature comforts," said Viv. "They wouldn't go and bust down a camping site in these thistles, nor would sheep."

A whirlwind or "willy-willy" was also ruled out for "if anyone has seen an old man whirlwind, they'd know that it doesn't stay in the one spot. It sweeps straight through a paddock and leaves a dread straight scar of knocked-down thistles, say, all heading in the same direction."

Thistles are a hollow-stemmed crop, and like oilseed rape, the stalks will not lie flat and remain flat when bent to ninety degrees. In experiments it was found that it is necessary to bend them in excess of ninety degrees and apply pressure. When this was tested, the stems simply snapped. Also the stalks bruise badly, and scars are visible if any mechanical weight is applied.

The accounts of circles or UFO nests in sugarcane are even more amazing. Having lived in Jamaica for twelve years, I am very familiar with the behavior of sugarcane. It reacts in a similar way to both thistles and oilseed rape, but grows considerably taller, to a height of eight to nine feet, and it is extremely heavy. What force as yet unknown to man could cause this gargantuan crop to bend to its will without causing any crop damage or broken stems?

Ron Gaist, a Sydney television executive, took aerial photographs of a diamond-shaped clearing in a cane field near Tully. A Queensland University study failed to find any explanation for the way the cane stalks had been pulled out by the roots and swirled into a mat about ten meters across, indicating the movement of some object. Willy-willies were again discounted, also crocodiles, "the 'nest' being too neat."

Another strange thing happened when the film was developed. "A bank of lights" appeared in several of the aerial photographs. Ron Gaist had no idea they were there until he had the film developed. The objects were not visible to the naked eye. Nor were they a fault in the camera because they did not appear on the rest of the film or in photographs taken before or since.

Ron Gaist also ruled out the likelihood that the markings were caused by sand ridges in the cane fields. "Sand ridges don't run in geometric patterns," he said. He believed he had uncovered new evidence of strange aerial phenomenon in Queensland's famed flying-saucer belt. "Now I'd like someone to tell me what I've photographed."

There is an Aboriginal legend that one of their gods, Chic-ah-Bunnah, was unlike the other gods, as he symbolized no other known living thing. He was shaped like a man. As he sped through the air he gave forth a blue light so dazzling no one could look upon him without being blinded. He ate glowing red coals and took off from the Earth with a frightening bang and a roaring noise.

Ron Gaist relates that an airline pilot has drawn up an electromagnetic grid system based on reported UFO sightings and that Tully lies at an intersection of this pattern. The belief that there is a connection between UFO sightings and flattened ground patterns is increasing.

In the UK in 1984 a design incorporating five crop circles suddenly appeared on the front page of a national paper, the *Daily Mail*. The reason for the unprecedented publicity was not so much the circles themselves but the celebrity of the photographer, Labor MP Denis Healey, now Lord Healey of Riddlesden.

Returning over the South Downs from his usual Saturday morning shopping in Seaford, East Sussex, he was amazed to see a single circle of about forty feet in diameter surrounded by four smaller circles equidistant from each other and the center of the circle. Then Mr. Healey, a well-respected amateur photographer, rushed home to get his camera and recorded the formation.

A few more formations appeared in the 1980s, but it was the 1990s that saw the appearance of many more circles and an increasing public interest in the phenomenon.

An interesting one in Warwickshire, on July 9, 2009, was the tetrahedron that was found with the apex of the tetrahedron pointing directly at the Chesterton Windmill near Hanbury. Famous as a landmark, the windmill has had a prominent position above the village for nearly 350 years.

Thought to have been built in 1632 by lord of the manor, Sir Edward Peyto, the windmill could have been designed by a pupil of Inigo Jones, John Stone. Peyto was a mathematician and astrologer, and as the windmill had a rotating top it is possible it might have been built as an observatory, with the rotating top acting as a station for Peyto's telescope. Later it became a working windmill grinding corn.

After giving my annual talk in Petersfield in October I was interested to meet one of Peto's (modern spelling) descendants who had been unaware of this forebear's links to the windmill and was delighted to know more.

Close by was the Radford circle. It now seems likely that unusual atmospheric conditions of lowered pressure are part of the process of the natural force behind this phenomenon.

CROP CIRCLE NUMBERS WORLDWIDE 2018

COUNTRY	CROP CIRCLES
Afghanistan	2
Argentina	12
Australia	199
Austria	14
Belgium	75
Bosnia and Herzegovina	1
Botswana	2
Brazil	35
Bulgaria	3
Canada	362
Chile	1
China	4
Colombia	2
Croatia	7
Cyprus	1
Czech Republic	231
Denmark	46
Egypt	3
England	3,668
Finland	13
France	58
Georgia	1
Germany	473
Hungary	25
India	5
Indonesia	4
Iran	1
Ireland	12
Israel	13
Italy	245
Japan	26
Kazakhstan	1
Kenya	1

COUNTRY	CROP CIRCLES
Latvia	4
Lithuania	1
Luxembourg	1
Macedonia	1
Malaysia	3
Mexico	16
Netherlands	480
New Zealand	18
Nigeria	1
Norway	41
Peru	4
Poland	86
Portugal	1
Puerto Rico	1
Romania	3
Russia	35
Scotland	12
Serbia	4
Slovakia	13
Slovenia	11
South Africa	7
South Korea	1
Spain	11
Sweden	24
Switzerland	79
Turkey	2
Ukraine	8
United States	433
Uruguay	1
Wales	13
Yemen	1
Total	**6,861**

Information courtesy of Bertold Zugelder

COMMENTS BY JAMES LYONS

The concept of Natural Healing in an environmental context is far from new. Most people can understand the magic of the countryside and Nature as a whole and its immense benefit to us and our physical, mental, and emotional being. We tend to consider the Sumerian period of around 400 BCE as a time of evolution of the Healing Arts. As we shall indicate, recent historical investigations have revealed a rather different perspective. This perhaps focuses more on the Yogic Period, circa 6000 BCE.

As far as science is concerned, this is truly the period in India revealing how Man and indeed all animals were an integrated evolutionary part of Nature. Yogic Science was the truly initiating factor that offers us a bridge from ancient to modern science. It is interesting to note that the first symbol of Man's connection to Nature is embedded in the Sri Yantra symbol. This nine-pyramidal emblem of Man's connection to Nature has only recently been resolved from a mathematical perspective.

The concept that the Cosmos was and still is the all-pervading, self-organizing field of energy is only now starting to be seen as the supposed Higgs field from which all material objects, including ourselves, emerge. This long-awaited perspective integrates ancient and modern science. Even the concept of the boson particle, which describes the nonmaterial world, is now beginning to be seen as the pseudo-particle, which accounts for the mental or conscious processes of the Cosmos.

As indicated in many places in this book, it is not the force of gravity that holds the Cosmos together, it is the electric force generated by spinning electric charges. These in turn are best modeled mathematically as closed standing waves around a virtual toroid. This in turn forms a dipole field not unlike a battery.

The Electric Universe model emerged from Hannes Alfven's research of the 1970s. It is these spiraling waves that interact with both halves of the brain and indeed with the auric shell surrounding the body. We owe it to Yogic Science for identifying the chakra systems of the body. It is not surprising therefore that crop circles mimic our body chakras as well as, at the cosmic level, the Galaxies.

Healing techniques based on concepts such as acupuncture, Hands-on-Healing, Reflexology, Reiki, Kinesiology, and so forth, are popular today since approved medical processes based on pharmaceutical products rely only on material techniques. The drug-based approach often has severe side effects, as we are well aware.

Crop circles are in fact the Earth's Chakra Systems, so being in a formation exposes one to the immediately local spiraling energies. These are essentially electrical in nature and most generally emerge from the Earth. As we are like sponges in the ocean, we are exposed to these columnar spiraling energies through our bodies. This is the same nonmaterial bosonic energy that our forefathers were most acquainted with.

Chinese medicine has embraced the idea of using the nodal points of the body as entry points for corrective insertion of appropriate signals. The whole process is somewhat like tuning an orchestra. If the body is harmonically tuned to a key frequency, then every body part plays its part in tune. A healthy person is one tuned to a common frequency.

We all know that orchestras need to tune up prior to a concert. In these days it is the oboe that holds this task. The realignment to a frequency of 440 Hz remains a bone of contention. The earlier Vivaldi period tuned at the slightly lower frequency of 432 Hz. This difference is noticeable to a learned audience. There is no doubt that the tuning of the spiraling columnar energies emerging from the Earth resonate with the cells of the body.

We should conclude this section with the observation that our forefathers, way back beyond the Yogic Era, were well aware of Earth healing. In recent years it has been discovered that natural volcanic hills have a common conic geometry, leading to pyramidal forms whose geometry relates to the Golden Ratio. One of these, the Bosnian Pyramid of the Sun, possesses many in-built tunnels showing healing properties. The British Museum analysis of organic remains in these tunnels revealed an occupation date of 34,000 BCE. Thus the healing properties of such structures have a long history.

Human interaction with the Earth's ambient energy fields dates to thousands of years before our recent turning to the healing properties of Earth Energies. We are at long last beginning to understand how the frequency spectrum of ambient vertical energies can have dramatic effects on our health, both good and bad.

11

CONCLUSION

This Elusive and Timeless Enigma

All truth passes through three stages. First, it is ridiculed. Second, it is violently opposed. Third, it is accepted as being self-evident.

ARTHUR SCHOPENHAUER (1788–1860)

I WONDER WHAT HAVE WE LEARNED as we have continued our journey through these examples of crop circle healing and its associated mysterious horizons? Has this multilayered phenomenon spoken to us, and on what path might it be leading us? Can we say that, as a result of our current understanding of this unique phenomenon and its events, and as our research continues apace, it has contributed to the development and expansion in certain new aspects of science?

Indeed we have come to understand more about the physics of the Universe and how they function and interact with the electric world in which we live and of which crop circles are a part. This is a phenomenon that rattles the brain, leaving an indelible impression on our psyche.

I am very aware that my knowledge and broad understanding have outpaced any previous learning of the past twenty-five plus years. Over the twenty-five years in which I have been involved in my "hands-on" investigations in this subject, I have become aware that it is a subject of scholarship, incorporating all branches of learning—ranging from all the sciences, music, farming, theology, history, ancient wisdom, customs, traditions, geography, and last, but certainly not least, art. How far one wants to venture into this university of endless and fascinating information and wisdom is entirely a personal matter.

Unexpected doors and windows have been opened in my brain and mind—sometimes taking me by complete surprise as a sudden realization of understanding bursts through into my consciousness.

Hopefully this book has answered many previously unanswered questions regarding this elusive and timeless enigma expanding our horizons and leading us on to further investigation.

However, as the river of time has flowed by, I have now reached the conclusion that there are things that can never be fully explained. When I was very young, so young that I could not yet read, I was shown a book in which there were marvelous colored birds with trailing feathers and adornments such as I had never seen before. On enquiring I was told that they were Birds of Paradise. "Are they real?" I asked. "Yes, they are real," was the reply. "Where is Paradise?" Answer came there none.

My sister and I didn't see much of our parents (as was usual in those days), except for an hour in the evening when we were spruced up and taken downstairs to the library. We were in awe of our parents, and so this was the most nerve-racking part of our day, and it took me several visits before I was able to summon up enough courage to ask my parents if they knew where Paradise was. Again, no answer. This was a severe disillusionment, as I had firmly believed that grown-ups knew everything, and this was the third time a grown-up had not been able to give me the answer. So I resolved that when I grew up I would find Paradise and take everyone there to see the exquisite and mysterious birds! My second fascination was with the Loch Ness monster, followed by Einstein's Theory of Relativity; next came Infinity. This was a real problem, and for many years I simply couldn't understand why at some distant point in time and space Infinity did not become Finite! AND then came the crop circles—what a bother they were, almost the worst of all, and how were we ever going to find out about from whence they came and who or what was the originating force behind them?

Now, after years of questioning, searching, and researching, I have realized that despite our knowledge of this subject having increased quite exponentially, there are certain questions—including those about crop circles—that can NEVER be properly answered. I have become perfectly content that there is an elusive, ineffable quality to them. Having realized this, and being quite comfortable with this realization, Infinity and other conundrums no longer bother me! What a relief!

A learned friend of mine wrote, "People travel the world to see the crop circles. Crop circles are the biggest thing that most people never experienced; a historic phenomenon. In a future time, people will look at these and wonder why they weren't headline news in our time—but then, we live in a strange and mad time, and many of us believe that the formations, and the energy fields inside them that can't quite be encapsulated in photos, point to another time. A time when we will understand them, using the archive records."

COMMENTS BY JAMES LYONS

Turning to conclusions, it is now becoming obvious that mainstream science is changing rapidly. There is considerable recognition that the current assumptions about such things as the Big Bang, Dark Matter/Energy, and so forth, are severely flawed. Gravity is a leftover force when the main source of energy, electricity, is balancing out its positive/negative charge.

The Electric Universe model is growing rapidly in significance. The latest work was presented recently in the Electric Universe Forum. Now we have exoplanets, that is, Solar Systems that are nothing like ours. The planets are still jumping orbits, so we have, for example, Jupiters located in orbits like Mercury.

What we are learning from crop circles is enormous. This includes the relevance of the geometries, the creation process, namely toroidal vortex flow, and, highly applicable to this book, the energy's frequency harmonic structure and its relation to spiraling subtle energies (left/right brain) and, most specifically, the brain frequency structures that are key to healing.

The two key words are *implosion* instead of gravity, which has everything to do with columnar vortices, and *cymatics,* which are responsible for the combination of frequencies determining patterns.

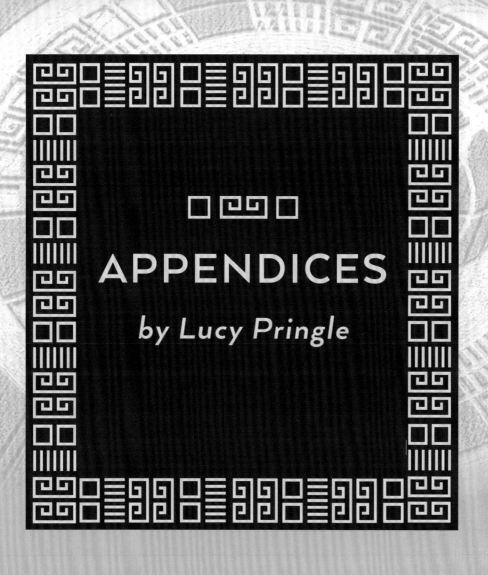

APPENDICES

by Lucy Pringle

EYEWITNESS ACCOUNTS

The nature of God is a circle of which the center is everywhere and the circumference is nowhere.

EMPEDOCLES (490–430 BCE)

OVER THE YEARS THERE HAVE BEEN relatively few credible reports of people actually witnessing crop circles being formed. Many people have claimed they have seen these events, but on closer scrutiny, their stories have not been substantiated.

However, there are four accounts that have successfully withstood critical examination, and these are included here for the readers' interest.

The first event took place in the Lincolnshire fen land in 1947. Frederick Smith was working on a farm.

> I was eighteen at the time. The month was April and the weather was very good, just nice and a gentle breeze with no planes in the air at the time.
>
> Suddenly a sound like "the gentle humming of bees" was heard. When the circles were laid down the noise was a high-pitched buzz, which seemed to come from far away. The circles were formed in about three minutes. I felt faint, and then passed out.

When Frederick recovered some three hours later he found that the crop of green oats, only six or seven inches high, was already rising up undamaged.

For Frederick to have fainted for so long would seem to indicate a rapid loss of air pressure surrounding him as when an airplane has to dive sharply and oxygen masks are needed.

GIANT PASTRY CUTTER

The second account comes from retired aircraft engineer Ray Barnes. In addition to being possessed of a logical and analytical mind, Ray is also a keen observer of Nature.

One afternoon he was going for one of his regular walks above the town of Westbury, Wiltshire, to a field where over the years he has witnessed many strange events taking place.

On this particular day, July 11, 1981, while walking his dog after a thunderstorm, Ray reports:

My attention was first drawn to a wave or line coming through the cereal crop. After traveling across the field in an arc, the "line" dropped to the ground and radially described a circle in a clockwise direction in approximately four seconds.

There are several points to make about the line.

(*a*) It was invisible.

(*b*) There was absolutely no wind, and the line exhibited no fluid tendencies, that is, the speed was constant, no wind waves before or after it.

(*c*) The line just appeared; there was no disturbance of hedge or trees at the field boundary.

(*d*) Estimated speed of the line was about 50 mph.

(*e*) There were no visual aberrations in front of, above, or behind the line.

(*f*) The line almost disappeared where the ground dipped, so it would seem the line was maintaining a constant height irrespective of ground contour.

(*g*) The crop heads only "jiggled" not bent, which would seem to indicate that the line had holes in it like the teeth of a giant comb or that the line was sufficiently weak for the cereal heads to pop through it when the pressure on them reached a certain level.

Barnes tells us that the circle was described *radially, not diametrically,* and at a constant speed.

The circle was executed in a single sweep. "The peripheral speed of the circle seemed to be about twice that of the line/arc speed. The crop in the circle went down as neatly as if it had been cut by a giant flan cutter. There was absolutely no spring back, which was rather awe inspiring as, if you watch a tractor crossing a field, there is always some spring back of the flattened crop."

Barnes subsequently developed an unusual form of cataract that he attributes directly to observing the crop circle appear.

WE FELT TINGLY ALL OVER

The third event took place on the outskirts of Hambledon, a small village in Surrey, on the evening of Thursday, May 17, 1990.

Gary and Vivienne Tomlinson had been for one of their regular walks up to the top of Byrony Hill. It was an unusually humid day—hot and sticky—and evening was approaching, and the Sun was setting. The air was still as they walked down the hill and across the fields toward home.

It was not until they were crossing the second wheat field that they noticed the wind blowing the crop. Looking back toward Byrony Hill the wind was so strong the trees were bending over. In a matter of seconds a mist appeared and rolled down the hill into the field where they were standing. It was like a shimmering whirlwind. They could hear the noise of the wind, intensifying to a high pitch like a set of panpipes. The noise was so great they looked up to see if a helicopter was overhead.

Suddenly there was a gust of strong wind pushing us from the side and above. The shimmering air circled around us. It was forcing down hard on our heads. We could hardly stand upright. Yet we also felt as if we were being sucked up at the same time. There was tremendous pressure both from above and below. We both felt tingly all over, like pins and needles from head to foot.

I tried to break free from the grasp of the whirling air but found myself trapped. I looked toward Gary; his hair was standing on end [Gary tells me that Vivienne's hair was also standing on end]. I tried to call out to him, but my voice seemed to get lost in the volume of noise as we were spun and swirled around. Suddenly the wind scooped us off the path into the wheat field. We took a great buffeting. It was very frightening.

Looking down we saw a circle being formed around us. It happened so quickly; it only took a couple of seconds. A spiral appeared anticlockwise and grew outward from the center. [Vivienne estimated the circle to be about two meters in diameter.] In the center of the circle there was a small pyramid of wheat, the stalks stacked up against each other. The whirlwind split into two, one going with a whir into the distance, skimming over the top of the wheat as it went. A second whizzed past me to one side, pushing down the wheat and then forming a second circle a little further away. This again only took a few seconds. We looked around for the first circle and could still see it like a light shimmering mist as it zigzagged into the distance over the top of the wheat.

Interesting things were happening in the circle in which we were standing. Miniature whirlwinds were appearing one after the other, small, glistening vortices perhaps four inches apart. They whirled around the wheat in small bunches toward the perimeter, gently laying the crop down and enlarging the circle. There was no wind now, and it seemed strange watching these shimmering whirlwinds as they spun around. They seemed to increase in number. We both looked toward the second whirlwind; it looked like a transparent glowing tube stretching up endlessly into the sky.

The sunset was beginning to fade. I turned my attention back to the miniature whirlwinds. They seemed to have lost their misty look, now appearing more like watery glass with a quivering line inside. They wobbled slowly, still running along the wall of the circle. There also seemed to be fewer of them. It was growing dark.

I panicked, grabbed Gary's hand and pulled him out of the circle. Slowly we made our way back in silence, stunned by the event. My ears ached, and we both felt lethargic and nauseous and were suffering from shock.

Neither Gary nor Vivienne were wearing watches at the time. They estimated the duration of the episode to have been approximately seven minutes, whereas it seemed to last an eternity.

Vivienne's ears were so painful that she visited her doctor, who diagnosed perforated eardrums.

There is little doubt that witnessing a crop circle appear before your very eyes is a traumatic event.

THE STONEHENGE JULIA SET 1996

This most remarkable event only came to light thirteen years after it had happened. It is noteworthy for several reasons; a pilot flying a light aircraft from Exeter to Thruxton flew over the field opposite Stonehenge on the afternoon of Sunday, July 7, with a passenger taking photographs, at which time the field opposite on the A303 was unmarked. The pilot disembarked at Thruxton, completed the necessary landing and flight forms, refueled, and then got back into the same plane to fly back to Exeter. To his great surprise when flying over the same field opposite Stonehenge some forty to fifty minutes later he observed an enormous formation measuring 915.2 by 508 feet imprinted in the wheat below. A gamekeeper and a guard at Stonehenge both confirmed that it had not been there that morning.

The formation was named the "Julia Set" as it represented complex computer-generated fractal image to the mathematicians, to musicians a base clef, and to marine biologists the cross-section of a nautilus shell.

Veteran researcher Colin Andrews related how the formation was first spotted from an aircraft at 6:15 p.m. The pilot crossed over the field with a passenger (a medical doctor taking photographs) at 5:30 p.m.

There was nothing in the field at that time but

when the pilot returned at 6:15 p.m. he saw the formation in the field. At about the same time (6:30 p.m.) his previous passenger drove past Stonehenge to see cars pulled off the side of the busy road.

When I interviewed the Wiltshire police I was told that the police emergency lines received several 999 calls just before 6:00 p.m. reporting a large number of vehicles pulled off the road causing a hazard.

German researcher Andreas Mueller has also supplied some vital information as a result of having visited the formation shortly after its appearance. He had listened to a man he took to be the farmer telling a group of people that he had had farm workers working in the field mending the fence until approximately 5:30 that afternoon.

Surely this is one of the most important events in the history of the crop circle phenomenon, as rarely do crop circles appear during daylight hours.

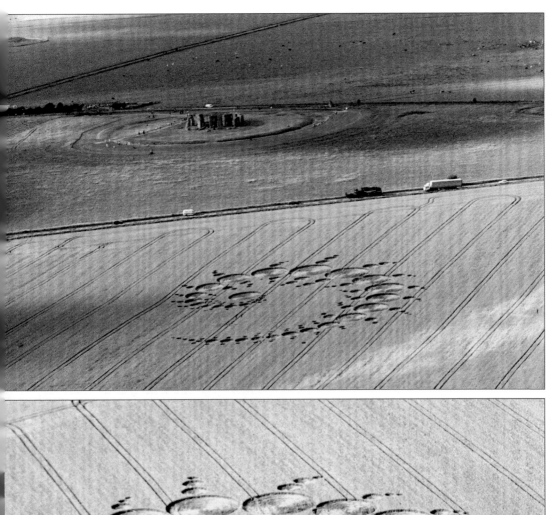

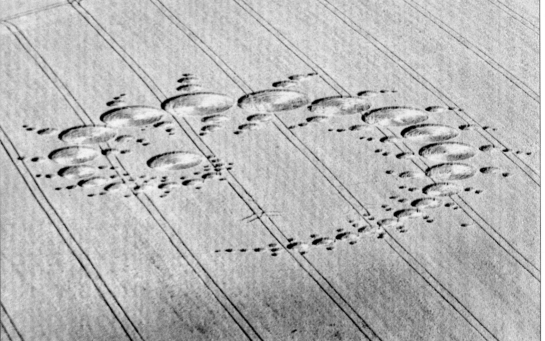

Fig. A1.1. The Stonehenge Julia Set, near Amesbury, Wiltshire, July 7, 1996.

THIRTEEN YEARS LATER

After giving a talk at Alton College in Hampshire in 2009, a friend telephoned me to say that someone she knew had been in a taxi and had told the taxi driver that she had just been to a fascinating talk on crop circles. (We will call the taxi driver M, as she was fearful of the publicity if her name were ever made public knowledge.) M replied, "I saw one appear opposite Stonehenge." Thinking she meant this year, my friend telephoned me but after making extensive inquiries, I realized that there was no circle anywhere near Stonehenge. I was given M's telephone number and told her what I had heard. "O dear me, no, it was years ago." I mentioned that up to 2009, only three formations had appeared close to or opposite Stonehenge, 2002, 1997, and 1996. "It was 1996, as my son, who was in the army, was on holiday, and I was driving down to see him."

I eventually managed to arrange a mutually convenient date to meet M and get her story on tape.

M and Tim (her son's friend) were driving to Somerset in July 1996 to see her son who was in the army. Driving down the hill toward Stonehenge she saw a lot of cars pulled off on the grass verge on the A303 opposite the stones. She mentioned that when people see maybe two cars or more pulled in and looking down into the field, other cars stop and gradually the traffic builds up and more and more cars draw in to have a look.

As she drew nearer Tim said, "Mrs. M, there's a crop circle there."

A car drew out and she managed to pull into the empty space and got out and joined the crowd of other people who were also watching what was happening. There was an apparition, an isolated mist over it, and as the circle was getting bigger the mist was rising above the circle. As the mist rose it got bigger, and the crop circle got bigger.

> There was a mist about two to three feet off the ground, and it was sort of spinning around, and on the ground a circular shape was appearing, which seemed to get bigger and bigger, as simultaneously the mist got bigger and bigger and swirled faster.
>
> It was gradual and you are standing there and you are thinking what is going on and everyone is discussing it and more and more traffic is building up and everything and you just think that all the time you don't really realize what is happening and then you think then that's it and the thing is getting bigger and you are thinking of the beginning and end. But you don't

realize what you are looking at. I didn't understand what was happening.

The mist wasn't anything from the ground as there was a clear space between the ground and the mist. There was no wind and no dust [she is an asthmatic]. It was the strangest thing I have ever seen. It was a calm summer's day.

When I asked her how long she stayed looking at the event, she said it was hard to say, but maybe twenty minutes or so, but she couldn't say as she had lost track of the time as she could not believe what she was seeing and was watching the event, not looking at her watch. The mist was still there when she left but whether the formation was still expanding she couldn't say.

What color was the mist? Well it wasn't brown or blue or pink; it wasn't coming off the ground. And it didn't go far up into the sky.

I asked her, "Did you feel strange?"

I felt, My God, what is going on, look what's happening, are we going to see a leprechaun or the men from Mars or a Sputnik in a minute or something?

I asked M which date it had appeared she thought a bit and then took my pad and wrote Sunday, July 7, 1996. She said she remembered this particularly as being a Sunday; she was driving *against* the traffic. She asked me, "Why haven't you heard about this before? There were so many people watching what was happening, not just me. Why didn't the other people talk about it?"

Indeed it was only by chance that I got to hear about it some thirteen years after it happened due to a passenger in M's car who had been to my lecture!

M hadn't mentioned it herself except to her family and friends.

On leaving M, I was puzzled by the time element of approximately twenty minutes. I could not budge M on this; she was adamant and insisted that that was what she had witnessed, and nothing I could say would make her change her mind. The other three reliable reports I have had of people witnessing crop circles appearing have all quite independently mentioned that the circle took between four and twenty seconds to happen. So why had this one taken so long? Was it due to the fact the other circles had just been small single circles whereas this one was large and complex?

On returning home I immediately telephoned James Lyons who was particularly interested in the cloud hovering above the circle, which he had always felt was part of the formation's creative process. Regarding the time element he asked me to send him the measurements and number of circles.

> As a result of work conducted in the 1990s, it is possible to calculate the time a formation takes to appear based on the size and number of circles. The method relates to the Earth's gravitational and magnetic fields. This predicts a velocity of the resulting vortex filament of some 10 feet per second. The filament propagates not unlike a solar flare, repeatedly looping through the Earth's surface "embroidering" a gradually evolving pattern. To create the 151 circles in the 915.2-by-508-foot pattern would take of the order of twenty to twenty-five minutes to create.
>
> The descending force emits an electrical discharge, which releases bubbles from the underground aquifers, which rise up through the surface of the ground and patterns are formed. The anchor point of the force is always off center.

This aspect has been observed many times over the years in certain complex crop circles.

> These patterns develop like "embroidery," half above the ground and half under the ground in a sort of looping manner.
>
> There is significantly less pressure inside than outside, therefore there is a sort of sucking motion from inside which bends or "sucks down" the crop at the base.

This drop in pressure was also illustrated by a report I was sent by Lynn Jenkins of Obrenpovac, Serbia, when visiting a circle at Radford, Oxfordshire, in 2009.

> It was windy as I walked toward the circle. Once inside the circle there was no wind, although nearby trees were moving. It was also very warm inside the circle. The conditions were cloudy and windy.

The mist would appear to be as a result of cool water vapor rising from the aquifer [underground spring] beneath and behaves in a manner similar to what happens in the lab when electrical discharges are created through water and different patterns emerge on the surface. Mist forms a little distance from the triggering point, which would support what occurred in this case. M could see the circle growing. It is when the hydrogen atoms recombine that all this happens as this draws in ambient energy. This is where the excess energy appears from. As for height, it would be no higher than the radius of the formation created, and the mist cloud would grow as the formation grew.

However, the more complex patterns have additional information contained in the sphere and who or what presses the button to make these is not within our present knowledge or understanding.

Indeed not only does it appear that M was correct in every aspect but it also corroborates the report by the pilot, the guard at Stonehenge, and the gamekeeper. It was a truly remarkable event.

Why did M and the other people who witnessed this event not report it?

I suggest you put yourself in their place—while watching this extraordinary scene as a group is one thing but as soon as you drive away, maybe you could start to wonder if it had really happened at all, and you would have to be a very brave person to go into your local pub and tell everyone about it for fear of ridicule.

Many strange things happened to people visiting this formation, especially to those visiting the formation shortly after it appeared.

I visited it on July 9, 1996, and was strangely reluctant to enter, and some instinct made me turn back after walking halfway down the field. Two friends, who were with me, continued into the circle and experienced extreme nausea that only cleared after they walked some distance away from the formation.

More reports of nausea and severe fatigue were to flow in from visitors to the Julia Set.

Nausea and severe fatigue after 10 minutes [in the formation] until 8:00 p.m. that evening. I had to lie down and slept for two hours.

The most extreme account came from a young scientist.

Felt mentally flat, unable to think or remember what I had done minutes before. Felt very similar to feeling of intense ultraviolet radiation or gamma radiation, both of which I am familiar with as a molecular biologist working in that field. Experienced initial nausea. [The effect lasted] all day until I went to sleep. Several hours later [I] experienced intense physical well-being and mental clarity.

THE EFFECTS OF CROP CIRCLES ON OUR BRAINS

WHAT IS THE RELATIONSHIP BETWEEN crop circles and electromagnetic fields?

Many people are researching the damaging effects of the electromagnetic fields emanating from radio masts; also there is a growing amount of literature and research into the beneficial properties of pulsed EMFs (electromagnetic fields).

Genuine crop circles are not randomly placed; they adhere to strict geophysical principles. The planet has a crisscrossing network of lines, some of which act as power points in the landscape.

Beneath the surface of the Earth's crust there is almost as much activity as in the heavens. Things are constantly moving around, to a greater or lesser degree, scraping against and colliding with each other just as the tectonic plates grow and slide over one another, creating electromagnetic fields and releasing pent-up gasses as they jostle, resulting periodically in earthquakes or volcanic activity.

In addition, the enormous pressure on rock crystals produces powerful local electrical fields, measuring several thousand volts per meter. When this action occurs, "luminosities" may result.

Studies by Michael Persinger, a professor of psychology and neuroscience at Laurentian University in Sudbury, Ontario, led him to believe that there is a connection between earthquakes, electromagnetic fields, unusual brain activity such as visual hallucinations, and paranormal events such as UFOs.

Our ancestors understood and were sensitive to these "energies" in a manner that many of us have lost in this highly technical world. Small shrines often developing into churches and temples were built on such places—Stonehenge, Avebury, Chartres Cathedral, and the Pyramids to name but a few.

There is increasing scientific evidence allowing us to make a connection between mechanical failures and seismic activity. It has been noted that car accidents occur at notorious black spots shortly before an earthquake or volcanic eruption anywhere in the world. These black spots are almost invariably located on "energy" lines. The survivors will often report that a local, familiar, straight road suddenly had a sharp right-hand bend ahead, while others will report seeing a nonexistent tree just before the accident happened.

There is an emerging body of opinion based on over twenty years of field investigation coupled with mathematical modeling that now recognizes the nature of the forces involved in crop circle formation. We now understand that the basic effect is founded on longitudinal electric waves, consistent with related geophysical phenomena such as lightning discharges. It is this triggering effect that releases the stored energy from underground water sources. The result is that the crop is drawn down to the ground by localized below-ambient pressure. More details of this process are described in James Lyons's prologue, pages xv–xvi.

There is also a wealth of evidence from different scientific disciplines showing that "energy" lines affect us in many diverse and bizarre ways. How we react to these is individual in manner.

BRAINY BRAINS

The brain is the most complex organ in the human body and the least understood. It is the control center comprising a hundred billion nerve cells that respond to eddy currents, and their effect and stimulation will depend on where the energy enters and its amplitude (field strength).

The brain weighs approximately three pounds, and despite the fact that it is only 2 percent of our body weight it uses 20 percent of the body's oxygen. The brain has two hemispheres, and there is a crossover effect, the right brain controlling the left side of the body and vice versa.

There are three principal parts of the brain, the particularly sensitive brain stem, the cerebellum, and the cerebral cortex. Each of these three areas is responsible for specific functions and the control of different activities. The brain itself does not feel pain.

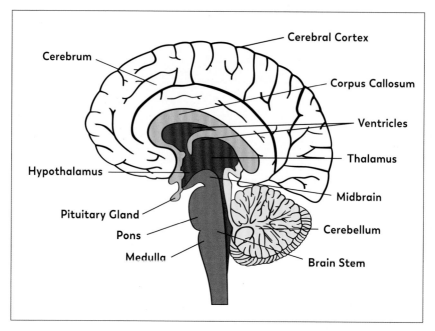

Fig. A2.1. The brain.

Do we only use 10 percent of our brains? How much of our brain do we use?

John Henley, a neurologist at the Mayo Clinic in Rochester, Minnesota, tells us that although it's true that at any given moment all of the brain's regions are not concurrently firing, brain researchers using imaging technology have shown that, like the body's muscles, most are continually active over a 24-hour period. Evidence would show over a day you use 100 percent of the brain. Even in sleep, areas such as the frontal cortex, which controls things like higher-level thinking and self-awareness, or the somatosensory areas, which help people sense their surroundings, are active.

Do our brains regenerate themselves? At one time it was thought that our brains could *not* regenerate. However, it is now understood that the neurons (nerve cells) in our brain are being constantly replaced and repaired naturally, even when we are adults. This process is called neurogenesis, and much research is being undertaken in this area, focusing with particular interest on sufferers of Parkinson's, Huntington's, and Alzheimer's disease.

Owing to the number of effects listed in the mental category, I am going to examine this aspect alone.

The part of the brain known as the brain stem is the area most affected by the majority of the following reports. The reaction to these effects, drawn from various sources of neurological literature, can be shown as a spike of between 18 and 18.5 Hz in the beta level of brain activity. The brain stem is located on the top of the spinal cord. It deals with important functions that keep us alive. It automatically controls our breathing, heartbeat, blood pressure, and circulation.

A PRESENCE

Below are several examples taken from responses to the questionnaires, letters, phone calls, and personal experience. We begin with the sense of a presence.

People often describe a place as having its own particular atmosphere, a distinctive quality unique to itself. In ancient days this was referred to as *genius loci,* an intelligent, protective spirit whose duty it was to live in and act as a guardian of the location. How it came to exist in a particular spot is conjectural; some suggest it was formed due to some magical event or as a result of energy lines. Could the genius loci be held responsible for the following report or was some other additional, unknown, and unseen quality present at the time?

A group of people from the Midlands visiting the 1993 Bythorn formation in Cambridgeshire were sitting and meditating in a circle inside the formation. The report sent in by one of the participants said,

> I sat next to John, and after a few minutes I was aware of someone walking up the tramline behind me and sitting down and joining us. Afterward, John turned to me, "Where is the person who sat down behind us?"
>
> John and I both independently heard someone approach but did not hear anyone get up and leave; the woman who had been sitting opposite us said that at no time had anyone joined the meditation.

The final area of discussion is "disorientation and memory loss" together with a lack of concentration and altered states of consciousness.

These effects outnumber all others in the questionnaire responses, and I believe they are due to a pull to the right cortex of the brain that is experienced by most people when entering a genuine formation. This pull makes performing any scientific task extremely difficult, as the concentration level and logical thought needed to accomplish the job is hard to achieve, let alone maintain for any length of time.

Many are the times that I have had to go back and repeat measurements and readings; and many are the reports I have had from researchers who have simply given in to superior odds and left their analytical work for another day. At times these effects also involve severe headaches.

In 1996, I decided to bury my bottles of water in a huge linear event named the DNA formation at Alton Barnes. Out of eighty-nine circles how should I select which ones to use? I found I was unable to count correctly beyond five. Time and time again, to the amusement of those present, I got to five but then jumped forward or backward out of sequence.

At last I realized what was happening: the "Inability to Count" syndrome that afflicts so many people when trying to count the stones within stone circles such as the Rollright stones in Oxfordshire where, to this day, I don't believe anyone has been able to count them correctly! I certainly haven't, despite trying on several occasions.

While inside the circle, Shelly Keel initially found that she was unable to draw the shape of the formation in her notebook.

> I couldn't get myself together enough to walk and draw the thing till just before we left. I had many goes at it but I just couldn't get it right. After about 1½ hours of trying I gave up for a while. When I drew it up just before I left, I realized I had been walking the same part over and over again. That was why I was unable to get it right. When I realized what had been happening it all came together quite easily.

In 1995 friend and colleague Keith Wakelam, a retired electronics engineer and author of many books, including *Discovering Eternity,* came with me to Wiltshire to help bury my small brown bottles of water.

It was a glorious early summer's day in June. We parked in the lane adjacent to the field and with the farmer's permission entered the field and made our way toward the formation.

MUDDLED MINDS

We entered the spiral, and then our problems began; we had the greatest difficulty finding our way to the center. Succeeding at last, I buried a bottle.

We were both using our dowsing rods, which behaved in a most strange and inexplicable manner that neither of us had ever previously experienced. Keith felt uncomfortable as though he was "being drained of his essential life force." I also started to feel very ill with the onset of a migraine (I am a migraine sufferer but now only get them when under extreme stress and that certainly was not the case that beautiful sunny summer morning). I started to feel sick and dizzy and experienced flashing lights. Keith was also getting worse and worse and was in a dreadful state. He too is an occasional migraine sufferer. He was experiencing flashing rainbow lights, his peripheral vision had gone, and he was feeling most unwell. We crawled out of the formation, and made our slow and halting way back to the car, where we sat like two heaps, unable to think or talk.

After a while Keith felt well enough to drive, he reversed the car and came back onto the main A40 Calne/Beckhampton road. It was not for a few minutes that I realized that something was amiss. I tapped Keith on the shoulder, "Do you realize you are driving on the wrong side of the road?" I asked.

We stopped for lunch at Stones restaurant in Avebury before attempting our familiar journey home. That was not so easy either; twice we got lost on the way back having taken a wrong turn. It was clear that we had lost all coherent thought, and we were thoroughly disoriented. Keith recovered after about twenty-four hours; I did not feel back to normal for several days.

Experienced crop circle researcher Christopher Bean was particularly taken with the 1999 Windmill Hill "Square."

I could not get the formation out of my mind until I'd got back to Bournemouth and had drawn it on graph paper. It took me three attempts to get what is in fact a rather simple formation onto the paper properly.

I had counted each circle in the formation and drawn it into my notebook in real time as I walked the lengths. I found that there was a rhythm between my counting each successive circle aloud and the steps I was taking. Between circles 12 and 13 on each side, I had to walk two to three steps before 13 and continuing on to 24 (the number of circles along the flanks). From this I knew there was a gap of standing crop halfway down each side, which the aerial shots have illustrated.

I could recite or recall the formation easily but this didn't stop me making countless errors when drawing it at home. I kept wanting 12 circles per side instead of 24. A full day later I realized what I was doing wrong and finally managed to draw it correctly.

LOST IN THE WOOD

I am much indebted for my final account to Norwegian Eva Haagensen, who once again describes a loss of time when going into crop circles.

I was in England last summer in different crop circles. I was in a group with John Gursli, and one in the group also had a PC. One evening John showed me a new crop circle. I felt a very, very strong energy from the picture on the PC. It was so strong that I could not look at it. It was a waving cross if you understand me. After I saw it on the PC I knew it was very important for me to come inside the crop circle.

John took us there the next day, and we went inside and I lay down inside it. After about twenty minutes I stood up again and I felt I had to go out again because it was so strong the energy that must have come inside my body. I went out and I decided to go back to our bus. But something had happened to me so I was not able to find the bus on the other side of a small wood. I went inside the wood to try to find the path. I do not know what happened to me in there because when I came out again I thought I had been there only a few minutes but it was an hour.

When I came out again I was totally alone. I saw nobody so I had to call for help from the others in the group. I was not able to find the way on my own. The strange thing was that I never before brought my telephone into the crop circles but this time something said I should bring it. So they found me, and I went back to the bus and I felt very strange. It was like I had a very heavy helmet on my head and that feeling was there the rest of the day.

After that I had a sort of energy in my head for five weeks that very often made me dizzy. I also want to tell you that I am a very sensitive person. I hope you can understand what I have written to you. My English is not perfect.

So what conclusion can we draw from these reports? It would appear that the combined effects of the residual electromagnetic energy found inside the circles together with the local geomagnetic activity are creating neurochemical reactions that are as yet not fully understood. Research is ongoing to determine the causes.

THE ASYRA TECHNIQUE (QEST4)

DIRECTOR MARK CONRAD LEADS the Asyra team. With a previous career in information technology, and ten years' experience at the helm of NutriVital Health, his role brings together the combination of energy medicine pioneer, natural health clinic, and nutritional products company that stands behind our unrivalled experience in this field. He writes that:

The Asyra software contains digitally-encoded information relating to a wide range of mental, physiological and emotional factors. The signals are output by the Asyra hardware as electromagnetic signals during testing. Using a simple and safe low voltage circuit formed by holding two brass cylinders, the response of the body to those signals is recorded. The response being measured is small changes in the electrical resistance of the skin. This information is relayed back to the software.

Running an Asyra test is an example of a process that we call bio-energetic testing. Bio-energetic (or just "energetic") testing is effectively "asking the body a question" and obtaining the response directly from the body's own physiology, without engaging the conscious and language centres of the mind.

The functioning of the human body is governed by informational signals. Some of these, such as the instructions for making proteins encoded in DNA are recognised by modern science. The epigenetic factors—how our experiences in life affect gene expression—are just beginning to be understood. It is likely that there are many other communication mechanisms at work that have yet to be explained scientifically. Biology is a very young science. The existence of control mechanisms beyond genetic determinism is not seriously disputed by modern science, but its implications have not filtered through to medicine in practice. This is a result of resistance to change and because it is not yet clear how to employ the knowledge in systematic treatment programmes. When we obtain responses from a bioenergetic testing device, the information is a mixture of commentary on the physical, chemical, emotional and mental state. Indeed, part of the skill of the practitioner of bioenergetic testing is to consider the information that comes from the system and decide how to recommend an individualised health and wellness programme.

Is the Asyra a diagnostic device? "Diagnosis" is derived from a Greek word meaning to "discern or distinguish." Asyra testing does indeed "discern" only in that it records a completely individual set of responses to signals. This may assist a holistic practitioner in the approach that is characteristic of such disciplines: "treating the patient, not the disease." Information obtained may support you in making a traditional diagnosis, if that is something you are trained and licensed to do.

The one definite and unchanging aspect of interpreting the test results is as follows: if an item shows up as unbalanced (usually a red or yellow indication against the item in the displayed list), then that signals that among the potentially hundreds or thousands of items tested, the body gave an above or below average electrical resistance response.

In different words, the body-mind system has indicated some kind of reaction to the item being tested, and along the lines of homeopathic treatment, we can use that to "remind" the organism to improve that particular aspect of homeostasis.

Consider a parallel from immunology: introduction to a pathogenic microbe initially causes a disturbance to the body, perhaps quite a serious acute reaction. However, as the information is relayed around the immune system, the body learns to cope with that particular pattern better next time.

The Asyra test is identifying items to which the body/mind system can learn better adaptive behaviours. These items may be as diverse as foods, pathogens, emotional patterns, colours or nutritional and pharmaceutical agents.

https://www.facebook.com/asyrasystems
https://twitter.com/AsyraUK
mark.conrad@nutrivital.co.uk

APPENDICES

by James Lyons

GRID LINES

WE NEED TO EXAMINE THESE electrical spiraling grid lines in a little more detail. The centerlines are double helices possessing a spiral angle of 36 degrees. They are, in fact, double helices resembling Slinky toys with adjacent spirals moving in opposite directions. This arrangement is just like the DNA within every cell of our bodies.

Where they cross over, a third, similar vertical spiral emerges. This is the centerline of a wider column of again spiraling energy, which aligns with the external circle of the acupuncture spider's web pattern.

Outside this central line system are single directional spiral lines, again Slinky-like but having a spiral angle relative to the line's flow direction of arc-sine (1/3) = 19.471 degrees. This type of line is called a tetrahelix line, first discovered by Buckminster Fuller. In church architecture, these often form the lines defining the edge of the church transept. These are the type of lines that reverse flow direction at Solstices and Equinoxes.

Outside these lines are the edge lines, usually one-half the distance from the centerline to the tetrahelix lines. These outer lines are, in reality, the location of the tube of energy in which these line structures occur.

It has already been stated that electricity flowing within the Earth can be relatively easily measured. In fact a simple digital voltmeter connected across two probes of differing metal such as brass and iron will register a few volts.

Perhaps more convincing is to dowse the tetrahelix lines to find a null point, that is, a point where there is no apparent source of current and where the battery's presence cannot be detected. Move it just a few inches in any direction and not only its presence is revealed but also its conical vortex.

Electrostatic voltmeters are often used in crop circles, but knowledge of the spider's web pattern and associated energy lines is needed to reveal the intricate underlying skeletal energy structure. All this knowledge has been lost by modern-day architects despite it having been known for thousands of years.

TELLURIC CURRENTS

A TELLURIC OR EARTH CURRENT is an electric current that moves underground or through the sea.

Telluric currents result from both natural causes and human activity, and although discrete, these currents interact in a complex pattern. The currents are extremely low frequency and travel over large areas at or near the surface of the Earth. Telluric currents are phenomena observed in the Earth's crust and mantle. In September 1862, an experiment to specifically address Earth currents was carried out in the Alps near Munich.

The currents are primarily geomagnetically induced. They are induced by changes in the outer part of the Earth's magnetic field and are usually caused by interactions between the solar wind and the magnetosphere or solar radiation effects on the ionosphere.

Telluric currents flow in the surface layers of the Earth. The electric potential on the Earth's surface can be measured at different points, enabling us to calculate the magnitudes and directions of the telluric currents and hence the Earth's conductance.

These currents are known to have diurnal characteristics wherein the general direction of flow is toward the Sun. Telluric currents will move between each half of the terrestrial globe at all times. Telluric currents move equatorward (daytime) and poleward (nighttime).

APPENDIX 6

DOWSING

THE ENERGY STRUCTURE of the Cosmos is such that when it manifests matter, it does so using just a few processes but in a very elegant way, such that the cosmic structures we are familiar with can be readily dissected to reveal their overall construction. This applies from the subatomic world up to galactic structures.

However, when we consider living matter we are invoking both mind and matter working in harmony.

The Cosmos is formed of billions of structures we term Galaxies. They congregate around nodal points in space, which resemble whirlpools in terms of function and are so-called Black Holes.

All Galaxies are connected. The energy field that permits this is electric in nature and is in the fourth, or "plasma," state of matter. It represents well over 99.9 percent of the matter in the Cosmos. We are familiar with the plasma state in the form of, for example, lighting in kitchens and supermarkets.

Plasma is composed of atomic matter in a separated state, that is, the particles of electric charge "float" around the nucleus of the atoms they are associated with.

In the Cosmos, all Galaxies are linked by networks of filaments of free electrons, which form helical structures across space. These filaments are termed Birkeland currents. They form networks of filaments not unlike a form of roadway system in which roundabouts are Galaxies and the connecting roads are Birkeland currents, slinky-like structures identifying a central line of the road as well as its gutters and grassy edges.

Galaxies, when mature, create conical spiral structures emerging from the galactic center. These arms contain Solar Systems, making ours but one of billions.

These same Birkeland filamentary structures surround the Earth and create the magnetosphere. It is not surprising therefore that a similar network of electric filamentary structures was involved in the creation of the Earth itself. Thus the Earth too is electric with a network of what we term telluric currents within and below the Earth's surface.

Since, as mentioned, dowsing can readily detect anything that spins or rotates, it has no problem detecting this road-like network of current. Humankind has known this for millennia.

These underground currents interact with all animals, including ourselves, only if we ask for a link. This is the basis of dowsing. Distance is no object in dowsing, but we must be extremely pedantic as to what we ask. The process is analogous to finding a specific word in, say, a book. If we have the right book, we next ask for the chapter, then the page number, then the paragraph, then the line, and finally we can hone in on a word, say, the name of someone.

Since the Earth's surface is in reality a hologram, we have in principle no problem finding what we need. The crossover points of these line networks, oriented to magnetic north and running north-south and east-west on the Earth, occur in a two-dimensional mimic of a Galaxy. We call these Spiders' Webs since they most often consist of six nested circles with eight radial lines. All of Britain's thirteen thousand medieval churches were built on these crossover points, and usually the altar is located over the point. All this knowledge has been largely lost; modern church architects plead ignorance of this most ancient knowledge. Needless to say, all stone circles are built on these nodal points.

These networks of lines are produced below the Earth's surface by an energy source, which is triggered by an electrical discharge from above. The bubble of energy, toroidal in shape, breaks through the surface acupuncture point. When the toroid—rising like a hot air balloon that has lighter air within it than outside it—breaks the surface, it collapses (implodes) in a very organized fashion, thereby drawing down the crop in its characteristic swirl of simply a circle.

How do we dowse this? It is just like dowsing a church or stone circle; we respond to the stored spin energy that created it all. By programming our thoughts we can even focus on one stalk of grain, indeed one seed, if we so desire. As in auric healing, some trained healers can determine what is wrong with us by our aura; we, in dowsing the crop, can measure the auric size of each seed if we need to. We now have a mathematical method whereby we can convert such readings into real energy measures such as joules per cubic meter.

In summary, humans, by means of their spiral DNA structure, which possesses the same helical angle (36 degrees) as we find in Earth Energies, resonate with what we are investigating. We simply ask and withdraw the information we need. We have evolved to be in every part of the Cosmos informationally.

The spiraling energy is key to healing. It resonates with our DNA, which in turn links with every cell of our body. We are, in effect, tuning in to, say, the correct frequencies for Parkinson's syndrome. The ambient energy field penetrates every cell, selecting the frequencies needed. This is how dowsing works in general and the crop circle effect in particular.

MUSIC AND GEOMETRY

THE UNDERLYING HARMONIC STRUCTURE of crop circles is based on the diatonic scale. The fundamental concept of musical scales goes back to Pythagoras. He evolved a numerical table called the *lambdoma* that involved ratios based on the numbers 2 and 3. Modern mathematics uses this principle in so-called modulo-9 arithmetic. Unlike in school where we learn to count from 1 to 10, the mod-9 system counts from 0 to 9. In this more universal procedure, we also embody the number 1. Simply: $1 + 2 + 3 = 1 \times 2 \times 3 = 6$.

Thus the two basic concepts we learn, namely arithmetic and multiplication, unite at the number 6.

This occurs everywhere in, say, chemistry. Thus, it is not surprising to find that the latest material to appear—graphene—is a carbon ring with 6 sides, the hexagon. We are now finding that this simple approach of the sequence 0 1 2 3 4 5 6 7 8 9 contains key numbers 3, 6, and 9.

Whereas the number 2 describes the material world and matter, the number 3 describes the mind world. This approach unites everything in science from Galactic levels down to subatomic levels such as the 3 quarks making up a proton, the basic unit of the quantum world.

Thus we begin to see how number can yield geometry. In music it is the diatonic scale that prevails. Our brain waves start to become noticeable at around 8 Hz. Why is this? It is simply that light propagates around the Earth at just under 8 Hz (7.83 Hz). If we investigate brain-wave frequency when, say, dowsing, the wave band spreads from approximately 8 to 14 Hz.

This lower limit is termed the "Schumann resonance." So starting at this frequency and going up in octaves, we have 8, 16, 32, 64, 128, 256, 512, and so on. Now, it just so happens that 256 Hz is middle C, known to all piano students. The octave with its eight white notes divides the frequencies into harmonic ratios. On the piano, these are tuned to equal temperament, which means dividing the scale into equal ratios with the lower note being 0.891 the frequency of its neighbor.

The key number of the Cosmos governing all materialized forms is 2. In music this is termed the octave, which is found at cosmic and quantum levels. Thinking of the octave on a piano keyboard, we know that between the notes C and upper C of the octave there are twelve semi-tones, the seven whites and five black notes. The frequency ratio of the adjacent semi-tones is 1.0594 corresponding to a tone ration of 1.12233445566. . . .

We find that the number 2, along with its companion prime number 3, is found everywhere in the Cosmos, from the largest galactic structures down to the quantum scale. They govern all patterns in the living and material world and are present in the I Ching. It is therefore no surprise to find both numbers in the crop circle world.

We find this diatonic ratio scheme everywhere in crop circles when we measure the separation of adjacent lines or, indeed, the radii of nested circles. In passing, it is interesting to note that the familiar discus shape of some mature Galaxies retains this fundamental ratio in successive rings. Indeed, simply dowsing the energy pattern around a common object such as a pepper pot on the kitchen table yields the same harmonic structure.

The result is that the diameter of the overall dowsable geometry of any common object shows that its ring-structure diameter is some nine times that of the dowsable aura of its central sphere.

There are so many other properties of the musical scale to be identified. Perhaps the most important one is the ratio of C to A, a so-called major sixth. Again we see the importance of this number. This note A is used to tune orchestras, with the first oboe undertaking the tuning procedure. Before 1953, this note was 432 Hz—note that the numbers add to 9. This tuning was defined by the mezzo-soprano/soprano voice range dating back to the era of Vivaldi and Verdi and the rise of opera.

What is so important is that this value is a key number in Quantum Physics. Division of 432 by a small correction to Pi, the ratio of the circumference of a circle to its diameter, yields the famous number the Fine Structure Constant, which for reference has the value 137.036. It has everything to do with waves traveling in a spiral motion in a circle, which is the basic way that crop circles are formed.

THE WILTON WINDMILL

The Wilton Windmill formation embodied a unique feature verifiable as a key element of mathematics. Unlike the Pi formation of 2008, which embodied a key number we all learn at school, this one codified an equation.

Although the codes presented, namely the ASCII codes, used universally to transform one's keyboard symbols into a string of ones (1) and zeros (0), the errors displayed in the field presented a tantalizing puzzle. First there were twelve radial lines representing the codes of each of the equation's symbols, as seen in figure 5.6 on page 74 and in figure A7.1 below. It is seen that where there are code lines present, that line represents a 1 (one), and no line a 0 (zero). However, for each radial there is the complementary code (exchanging 1s for 0s and vice versa anticlockwise of each radial).

These lines form their own codes, which, in fact, are pure integer numbers ranging from 200 to 300-plus. It turns out that the average of these is 274 and this, it happens, is twice the number 137. As mentioned earlier, in Quantum Physics this is known as the Fine Structure Constant, arguably the most important number in this branch of science.

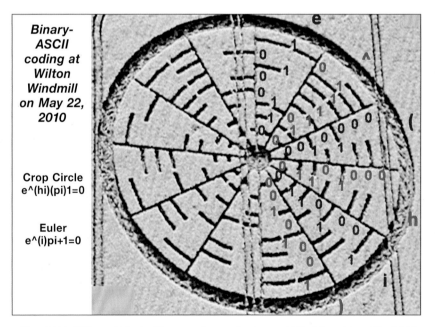

Fig. A7.1. Wilton Windmill, near Great Bedwyn, Wiltshire, May 22, 2010.

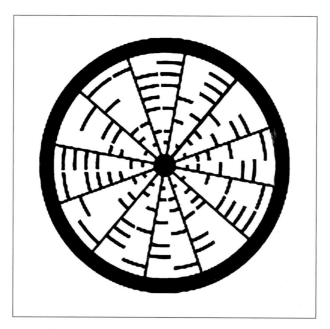

Fig. A7.2. A diagrammatic representation
of the Wilton Windmill crop circle.

Also, since there are eight symbols in an ASCII code, this reminds us of the diatonic scale (white notes on the piano), which we find everywhere in Earth Energies. Thus each radial has a left- and right-hand code (scale sequence) associated with it. Playing these "tunes" on the piano, however, did not turn out to offer very inspiring music!

A recognizable equation only emerges when its first symbol is aligned with the windmill. Reading the codes on the clockwise side of each radial reveals Leonhard Euler's famous Euler's Identity Equation, well known to mathematicians.

Within this equation one finds Euler's number having the value 2.7183. . . . In Earth Energy investigations the key number 2.72 feet emerges and is found throughout all ancient sites and crop circles. This length is known as the megalithic yard.

THE STONEHENGE JULIA SET

THE JULIA SET FORMATION (fig. A1.1 on page 205) is unique in several ways. Formed in July 1996, it was created on an Earth-acupuncture point in the same Earth Energy complex as Stonehenge itself. As noted, its midafternoon creation was in full sight of wayside observers who viewed the laying down in total of some 192 circles, starting from its center and spiraling outward toward its periphery. A cloud was observed to hang over the formation while the emerging pattern formed beneath. These observations in themselves confirmed the fact that crop formations were capable of being created by Mother Nature.

Photographic evidence later revealed the startling pattern that had been laid down. In principle, despite consisting of simple circles, the arrangement of the circles in both location and size revealed clearly the sequential fractal nature of the creation process. This is entirely consistent with what is seen throughout the Cosmos. The overall impression indicates a strong connection to music, resembling remarkably the universal bass clef symbol. It has been seen that throughout Nature reference to harmonic scales is widespread, being readily distinguishable through quantum to cosmic scaling. Again the diatonic scale is prevalent—in this case the relative scaling of adjacent circle diameters reveals this underlying process.

We are now in a position to describe the pattern formation in more detail based on the universal descriptions of the creation of toroidal waves. The overall formation is "housed" in a hemispherical dome whose walls are Langmuir double layers. This dome is created from the expanding shell of energy emerging from the initial discharge to the underground water blind spring. Within this is the expected toroidal ring having a central hole that defines the center circle of the formation. This in itself is a central columnar vortex reaching to the hemispherical energy shell above. This forms a Hannes current circuit as per the ubiquitous form found throughout the Cosmos. The toroid hosts a toroidal wave with a winding ratio of unity. Unlike a toroidal wave, which has a wave with a filament of constant diameter, this formation utilizes a filament, which is linearly conical in shape. It is this narrowing property that dictates the size of the individual circles decreasing in size as the spiral length increases. It is seen that for up to near one azimuthal rotation the major circles are decreasing as dictated by the conical "embroidery threading" vortex filament. Beyond this first 360-degree rotation, it can be seen that the sizes of the circles decrease in a linear progressive manner. This occurs since the conical vortex has reached its maximum diameter and starts to decrease in width, thus accounting for the progressive reduction in circle size. Thus the creation vortex filament is, in fact, of a very long biconical form. Its symmetrical form accounts for the overall spiral length. Since this structure is universal in all the plasma physics we see, it is more than comforting to find the Circle Makers using this same concept, thus indicating most explicitly the universal principles of cosmic construction.

We still need to address yet one more question, namely, the myriad smaller circles spreading on both sides of the main circle sequence. Studying again the toroidal wave model, it is the spirals-upon-spirals concept that gives the game away. These are the way in which we model higher-dimensional space. The idea was first observed by Leadbeater in his Theosophical studies of the universal atom mentioned earlier. In this case, for each major circle there are three smaller circles on either side. The farther away the circle is from its much larger host circle, the smaller it is. This overall arrangement indicates in two dimensions what we are seeing in the model in three dimensions. This clue to higher dimensions is crucial to our emerging understanding of higher dimensions in Quantum Physics, particularly the current key model describing higher-dimensional space known as M-Theory.

SUGGESTED READING

RECOMMENDATIONS
OF LUCY PRINGLE

Andrews, Colin, and Pat Delgado. *Circular Evidence: A Detailed Investigation of the Flattened Swirled Crops Phenomenon.* London: Bloomsbury Publishing PLC, 1990.

Antic, Ivan. *The Process of Realization.* North Charleston, S.C.: Create Space Independent Publishing Platform, 2017.

Arnold, Larry E. *Ablaze! The Mysterious Fires of Spontaneous Human Combustions.* New York: M. Evans, 1995.

Bartholomew, Alick, ed. *Crop Circles: Harbingers of World Change.* Bath, UK: Gateway, 1991.

Bobroff, Gary S. *Crop Circles, Jung, and the Reemergence of the Archetypal Feminine.* Berkeley: North Atlantic Books, 2014.

Brekkesto, Eva-Marie. *Crop Circles: History, Research and Theories.* Salisbury, UK: Wessex Books, 2011.

Broadhurst, Paul, and Hamish Miller. *The Sun and the Serpent.* Hillsdale, N.Y.: Pendragon Press, 1989.

Brown, Allan, and John Michell. *Crooked Soley: A Crop Circle Revelation.* Brighton, UK: Roundhill Press, 2005.

———. *Crooked Soley: A Crop Circle Revelation.* Squeeze Press (on-line publication), 2017.

Burl, Aubrey. *John Aubrey and Stone Circles: Britain's First Archaeologist from Avebury to Stonehenge.* Stroud, UK: Amberley Publishing, 2013.

Collins, Andrew. *The Circlemakers: Revolutionary New Vision of the Crop Circle Enigma.* Sydney: ABC Books, 1992.

Currivan, Jude. *The Cosmic Hologram: Information at the Center of Creation.* Rochester, Vt.: Inner Traditions, 2017.

Davis, Beth. *Ciphers in the Crops*. Bath, UK: Gateway, 1992.

Devereux, Paul. *Places of Power: Measuring the Secret Energy of Ancient Sites*. London: Blandford, 1999.

———. *Symbolic Landscapes*. Glastonbury, UK: Gothic Image Publications, 1992.

Glickman, Michael. *Crop Circles*. Glastonbury, UK: Wooden Books, 2005.

———. *Crop Circles: The Bones of God*. Berkeley: Frog Ltd., 2009.

Haslehoff, Eltjo. *Crop Circles: Scientific Research and Urban Legends*. Berkeley: Frog Ltd., 2001.

———. *The Deepening Complexity of Crop Circles*. Berkeley: Frog Ltd., 2001.

Hesemann, Michael. *The Cosmic Connection*. Bath, UK: Gateway, 1996.

Knight, Peter. *West Kennet Long Barrow: Landscape, Shaman, and the Cosmos*. Dorset, UK: Stone Seeker Publishing, 2011.

Kollerstrom, Nick. *Crop Circles*. San Antonio: Brunton Business Publications, 2002.

———. *Crop Circles: The Hidden Form*. Salisbury, UK: Wessex Books, 2002.

Meaden, George Terence. *The Circles Effect and Its Mysteries*. Wiltshire, UK: Artetech, 1989.

Michell, John. *The New View over Atlantis*. London: Thames and Hudson, 1986.

Moore, Judith, and Barbara Lamb. *Crop Circles Revealed*. Flagstaff, Ariz.: Light Technology, 2002.

Moulton-Howe, Linda. *Mysterious Lights and Crop Circles*. New Orleans: Paper Chase Press, 2000.

Pratchett, Terry. *Witches Abroad*. London: Victor Gollancz Ltd., 1991.

Pringle, Lucy. *Crop Circles: Art in the Landscape*. London: Frances Lincoln, 2010.

———. *Crop Circles: The Greatest Mystery of Modern Times*. London: Thorsons, 2000.

———. *Crop Circles: The Pitkin Guide*. London: Jarrold Publishing, 2004.

Sheldrake, Rupert. *Morphic Resonance: The Nature of Formative Causation*. Rochester, Vt.: Park Street Press, 2009.

Silva, Freddy. *Secrets in the Fields: The Science and Mysticism of Crop Circles*. London: Hampton Roads, 2002.

Thomas, Andy. *Introduction to Crop Circles*. Salisbury, UK: Wessex Books, 2016.

———. *Vital Signs: A Complete Guide to the Crop Circle Mystery and Why It Is Not a Hoax*. East Sussex, UK: SB Publications, 2002.

Wheatley, Maria, and Busty Taylor. *Discovering Wiltshire: A Gazetteer of Ancient Sites*. Marlborough, Wiltshire, UK: Celestial Songs Press, 2013.

Wilson, Terry. *The Secret History of Crop Circles*. Paignton, Devon, UK: CCCS, 1998.

Zollinger, Elizabeth. *Crop Circles: An Open Case*. Self-published, 2012.

RECOMMENDATIONS
OF JAMES LYONS

Beutel, Andreas. *Global Scaling.* Munich: FQL Publishers, 2008.

Coates, Callum. *Living Energies: An Exposition of Concepts Related to the Theories of Viltor Schauberger.* Dublin: Gateway Books, 2018.

Edwards, Lawrence. *The Vortex of Life: Nature's Patterns in Space and Time.* Edinburgh: Floris Books, 1992.

Ehlers, Gabriele and Stephan. *Global Scaling Theory.* Munich: Carl Harsen, 2009.

The Electric Universe. www.thunderbolts.info.

Schwenk, Theodore. *Sensitive Chaos: The Creation of Flowing Forms in Water and Air.* East Sussex: Rudolph Steiner Press, 1965.

Scott, Donald R. *The Electric Sky.* Portland, Ore.: Mikamar Publishers, 2006.

INDEX

Page numbers in *italics* indicate illustrations.

235

ABOUT THE AUTHORS

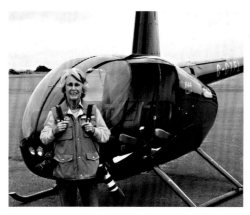

Lucy Pringle is one of the world's leading crop circle photographers. Her images have been used and continue to be used worldwide on TV, in films, books, and magazines, including on the *40th Anniversary Tribute Album to Led Zeppelin*. An exhibition of her aerial photography in 2002 was nominated the *Sunday Telegraph's* Art Critics' Choice.

Lucy was educated in England, France, and Switzerland and was a founding member of the Centre for Crop Circle Studies. She is widely known as an international authority on the subject, working with scientists from all over the world on the effects of electromagnetic fields on living systems, including the effect of genuine crop circles on Parkinson's disease.

She has been a guest on BBC and Meridian Television and the BBC World Service and has also appeared on William Gazecki's *Crop Circles: Quest for Truth* and the Discovery, Learning, and History Channels. She has lectured in France, Germany, Spain, Bulgaria, Canada, and Curitiba, Brazil, as well as in Chicago and Taos, New Mexico.

A member of the British Society of Dowsers, she is also the author of *Crop Circles: The Greatest Mystery of Modern Times* and *Crop Circles: Art in the Landscape*. She lives in Hampshire, England. Her website is **https://cropcircles.lucypringle.co.uk**.

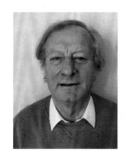

James Lyons is a chartered engineer, specializing in aeronautical research. Educated at the University of Birmingham (UK), James worked for 30 years in the aerospace industry, becoming chief engineer on new aircraft projects. He also worked for 30 years at the University of York (UK), primarily researching energy technology. He has been a visiting professor at several UK universities and is a member of the British Society of Dowsers. He lives in Yorkshire, England.